CHOOSING WISDOM

CHOOSING
WISDOM

STRATEGIES AND INSPIRATION
FOR GROWING THROUGH
LIFE-CHANGING DIFFICULTIES

Margaret Plews-Ogan, MD,
Justine E. Owens, PhD,
and Natalie May, PhD

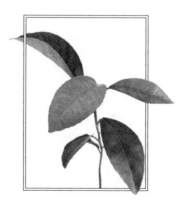

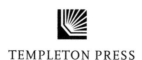

TEMPLETON PRESS

Templeton Press
300 Conshohocken State Road, Suite 500
West Conshohocken, PA 19428
www.templetonpress.org

The authors have protected the confidentiality of the physicians and
patients by describing their stories with altered identities and details, except
for the material featured in the documentary *Choosing Wisdom* and those
pain participants who released their interviews for public dissemination.
Quotes of physicians and patients have been edited for readability only.

Figure 1, © 2004 from "Posttraumatic Growth: Conceptual Foundations
of Empirical Evidence" by R. Tedeschi and L. Calhoun in *Psychological
Inquiry*, is reproduced by permission of Taylor & Francis Group, LLC,
http://www.taylorandfrancis.com.

Designed and typeset by Gopa & Ted2, Inc.

Library of Congress Cataloging-in-Publication Data
Plews-Ogan, Margaret, 1956-
Choosing wisdom : strategies and inspiration for growing through
life-changing difficulties / Margaret Plews-Ogan, Justine Owens, Natalie May.
p. cm.
Includes bibliographical references and index.
ISBN 978-1-59947-395-6 (pbk.) — ISBN 1-59947-395-X (pbk.) 1. Mental healing. 2. Wisdom. 3. Self-actualization (Psychology) 4. Physician
and patient. I. Owens, Justine. II. May, Natalie. III. Title.
RZ400.P76 2011
615.8'51—dc23
2011052610
Printed in the United States of America

12 13 14 15 16 17   10 9 8 7 6 5 4 3 2 1

Contents

Acknowledgments

OUR PROFOUND GRATITUDE goes out to the patients and doctors in the Wisdom in Medicine project and the *Choosing Wisdom* documentary who courageously and generously shared their stories. We also benefited greatly from the wisdom of our collaborators and advisors: Lawrence Calhoun, Monika Ardelt, Sigall Bell, Jo Shapiro, Tom Gallagher, David Morris, Danny Becker, Wendy Levinson, and Jim Childress. Special thanks to Martha Menard for helping us develop our database for the content analysis of the interviews. We offer our deepest appreciation to the John Templeton Foundation for giving us an opportunity to do this work. And of course to our editors, who first suggested this book and who walked us patiently through the process.

A special thanks to Richard Bell, professor of philosophy at the College of Wooster, who thirty years ago encouraged me to "pay attention to the sufferer" if I wanted to understand more about suffering. I am deeply grateful to my husband, Jim, a pediatrician whose vision and imagination inspired this project from the beginning, and whose love and wisdom kept me from straying too far afield. And to my children, Erin and William, who are a source of constant inspiration, joy, and hope for the world. —MPO

My heartfelt appreciation goes to my parents, William and Monica, and my son, Sam, three of the wisest people I know. —JEO

Thank you, Jim and Maddie. Every day you show me love and wisdom, and you inspire me to do the same. —NM

PART ONE

Background

We don't receive wisdom, we must discover it for ourselves after a journey that no one can take for us or spare us. —MARCEL PROUST

THE GUEST HOUSE

This being human is a guest house.
Every morning a new arrival.

A joy, a depression, a meanness,
some momentary awareness comes
as an unexpected visitor.

Welcome and entertain them all!
Even if they're a crowd of sorrows,
who violently sweep your house
empty of its furniture,
still, treat each guest honorably.
He may be clearing you out
for some new delight.

The dark thought, the shame, the malice,
meet them at the door laughing,
and invite them in.

Be grateful for whoever comes,
because each has been sent
as a guide from beyond.

—RUMI

1. Introduction

It All Began with a Question: "How Do They Do It?"

F ACING ADVERSITY is a common human experience, and I suspect that each of you reading this has faced hardship in your own life—some extreme, some less severe. I also suspect that you may have noted how you have been changed in a positive way—become a better human being—through the response to a difficult circumstance. You may know particular people who have lived through very difficult circumstances and whose lives, rather than exemplifying anger, bitterness, or disillusionment, manifest compassion, optimism, and strength. They seem to see the deeper meaning of things, to understand the bigger picture, to be able to tolerate life's ambiguities. The word "wise" might come to mind when trying to describe those who have faced difficulty and come out the better for it.

Until recently, much of the psychological literature on how humans cope with adversity has focused on its negative impact (posttraumatic stress), and much of the philosophical and religious literature has tried unsuccessfully to shed light on why humans suffer. But what about those people we all know who have grown and changed for the better in the face of harsh circumstances? How do they do it? What, exactly, have they learned about themselves and the world that helps them to be better human beings? The German philosopher Friedrich Nietzsche, who himself suffered a lifetime of physical illness, said, "What doesn't kill me makes me stronger." What can we do when we face difficulties in our own lives to help us grow stronger and perhaps even wiser because of those difficulties?

As a practicing physician, I* care for many patients whose illnesses I cannot cure and whose situations I cannot alleviate. Some patients move through those experiences and emerge with positive changes. They learn things, grow, and change in positive ways. *If I could not ameliorate their circumstances, are there nonetheless ways,* I wondered, *that I could help my patients to address these challenges that increased the likelihood that they would be changed for the better?*

I am also a patient safety expert. In that role I work with physicians who confront perhaps the most difficult experience imaginable in their professional lives: making a mistake that harms a patient. Physicians go into medicine to help people. When the opposite occurs, when something they do harms a patient, it cuts to the core of who they are as doctors and as people. Some physicians are able to move through this experience and emerge as better doctors, with increased humility and compassion, more mindful of their limitations and better able to see the bigger picture. How could we help physicians who face such circumstances to confront them in a positive way, one that increases their capacity for learning and that promotes humility, compassion, and the ability to see the bigger picture?

When I started down this road, I can honestly say that I had not spent much time thinking about the definition of "wisdom." But I have spent twenty-five years observing people who faced difficult circumstances and the positive changes that occurred as a result. When I began to investigate the various conceptualizations of wisdom, the parallels were striking: compassion, empathy, humility, understanding the deeper meaning of things, recognizing the limits of what we can know, a clear-eyed view of the world, seeing things from another perspective. I had witnessed people learning all these things from difficulties in their lives. The questions arose: Can adversity result in greater wisdom? If so, how can we foster growth and wisdom when people are coping with adversity? How did these exemplary people do it? What did they learn and how have they changed? If they can do it, can I? Can we help each other?

---

* Throughout the book, "I" refers to the primary author, Margaret Plews-Ogan.

That is the subject of this book. It is a book about regular people who faced difficult circumstances in their lives. It is built on the narratives and the findings of the Wisdom in Medicine project, a three-year investigation that examines two very different circumstances of suffering and two very different populations trying to cope with that suffering. These different groups (patients coping with chronic pain and physicians coping with having been involved in a serious medical error) were chosen for two reasons. First, they represent highly challenging circumstances in and of themselves, and our ultimate goal is to identify ways to help people cope positively with these circumstances. Second, despite their differences in perspective, we wanted to identify the common thread of change, illuminate the positive response to adversity in general, and understand more about how to help all people who face adversity in their lives.

Through in-depth interviews, the study investigators delved into how people respond to adversity, how they change, and what helps or hinders positive change. We also explored whether the growth they describe correlates with the components of wisdom. Investigators interviewed over 130 physicians and patients, and a common pattern has emerged, a path that traces the journey of coping with adversity and the commonality of what people see as their growth.

When people describe how the process of coping with adversity has changed them, what they learned, and how they do things differently, they use the language of wisdom. They describe how they are now more empathetic or compassionate; they have a wider-ranging perspective on things; they understand the deeper meaning of circumstances and events in their lives; they grasp the complexity, ambiguity, and uncertainty in life. They reflect on how they have grown in ways that they could not have if they had not struggled with this difficult circumstance, because their usual way of functioning had to change in order to cope.

Participants also describe a process or a journey through this experience. Many refer to this journey in the language of story, with low points and turning points, themes, and morals. They talk about what they had to let go of (perfection, blame), what they had to accept or acknowledge (limitations, ambiguity, imperfection), and what they had to do to move forward (accept responsibility, take charge). They talk about what it took to get them there (the support of colleagues, friends, and family; trying things; being open; sharing their story; forgiveness), and they have sage advice for others facing similar circumstances.

This book tells the stories of how ordinary people move through those experiences and emerge as better people, better doctors, with more compassion and empathy, and with a greater capacity to see themselves and situations honestly, stronger and more empowered, and wiser.

Although the two populations that were studied in the Wisdom in Medicine project may at first glance seem like strange bedfellows, their superficial differences in circumstance in some ways make it easier to focus on the common human experience of coping with adversity. I also believe that their unique circumstances are oddly universal. Who among us has not made a mistake and had that awful moment of realization? Who has not struggled with the guilt and shame that accompany the mistakes we make—big or small—and the resultant challenge to our deepest feelings of being a failure, a fake, or a sinner? I suspect that we all have felt some physical or emotional pain in our lives, and we can imagine the suffering that those patients must feel whose pain cannot be resolved.

The ultimate goal of this book is to enhance our understanding of how to help people who are facing challenges in their lives and to stimulate thought and conversation about how wisdom can be developed through these life challenges. Our hope is that by paying careful attention to the journeys of these exemplars we might shed light on how people can grow and change through adversity and how that contributes to the development of wisdom.

The people in this book are models of coping positively. Most of them have faced extreme difficulty. Patients endured continuous pain so severe that they could not eat or sleep, and they could not care for themselves or their families; some even contemplated suicide. Physicians, in most cases, were dealing with situations that resulted in harm to a patient: mistakes including a delayed diagnosis of cancer, failure to recognize infection that eventually was fatal, misdirecting a needle that resulted in puncture of an artery or a vital organ—all with devastating consequences. In some cases the physicians themselves contemplated suicide, stopped practicing, or found themselves at least temporarily unable to function. In many cases the "mistakes" were actually known complications of a procedure, but the physicians involved experienced them as a mistake. For many, it didn't matter if there was no discernible way to have prevented the bad outcomes. They still felt responsible.

We do not dwell on or describe in great detail the circumstances that these people faced. If you think about it, as humans we tend to grab hold of the details of tragedy and use those details to protect ourselves in some way from the thought that something similar might happen to us. Blame and judgment are ways we protect ourselves from our common vulnerability. As an example, I recall hearing about a tragic traffic accident that killed a teenage girl in my community, a girl exactly the age of my daughter. I was horrified, frightened, and so very sad. But I found myself searching for the details of the tragedy. Predictably, when I discovered that the accident happened on a road that my own daughter never traveled, my first insuppressible thought was, *Well, that won't happen to my daughter. She never drives that road.* The next thought was, *In fact, I would never let her drive that road.* My judgment, so swift and sure, came out of my deep desire to separate myself from other vulnerable mothers who suffer loss and grief, other humans who suffer for no discernable reason. I *looked* for a reason, assigned judgment, and thus protected myself from the truth—that this could happen to anyone. But when we set aside the specifics, we are more likely to be able to see and acknowledge the common experience of suffering and vulnerability and relate it to our own lives.

We want you, the reader, to be free to connect with the very common experiences of pain, or making a mistake, or misjudging a situation, or having to accept limitations of the body, and focus on the ways in which these people were able to move through their experiences and learn, grow, and change for the better. We focus on people's responses, rather than their specific circumstances, because in the responses to difficulty we can find the keys to developing wisdom in our own lives.

This book is arranged in three parts. Part 1 provides the conceptual backdrop for our understanding of how people cope positively with difficult circumstances. The first concept we tackle is wisdom (chapter 2). If you are like me, you may not have given much thought to the concept of wisdom, and even if you have, it is not something whose definition comes easily to mind. Wisdom is, however, something worth thinking about. In fact, as Stephen Hall puts it in his wonderful book on wisdom and neuroscience, "Thinking about wisdom forces you to think about the way you lead your life" (2010, 10). I hope this chapter stimulates your curiosity about this elusive but inspiring concept, because thinking about wisdom, in and of itself, is a worthy and productive endeavor.

The second concept we discuss (chapter 3) is an exciting and fairly new paradigm—one that has emerged in the last ten years and has had a dramatic impact on how we think about the effects of trauma. That is called posttraumatic growth. Much of the psychological literature prior to this had focused on the negative effects of trauma. Researchers and practicing psychologists Lawrence Calhoun and Richard Tedeschi, editors of *Handbook of Posttraumatic Growth*, noticed that there were people who seemed to learn and grow in positive ways in response to trauma and began to study that process. They and others began to research this phenomenon, which was a powerful first step in understanding how and why people respond positively to hardship. Eventually we may understand how to help people who face adversity.

In the second part of this book, we become keen observers and listeners as we recount the stories of people who have struggled with hardship and come through the experience better for it. The stories people tell have common elements or themes that are part of this journey, and we describe these as acceptance, stepping in, integration, new narrative, and wisdom. Part 2 is arranged around these themes. Not everyone's story contains each of these elements, and different journeys are dominated by different elements. It would not be accurate to describe these as linear steps, since people move back and forth, skip over, and repeat these elements in their journey. So we use the terms "elements" or "themes" to avoid the implication that this process is somehow linear. In fact, for most people, this process is quite iterative or circular. Rachel Naomi Remen, physician and author of *Kitchen Table Wisdom*, makes the point that this process of discovering wisdom is a dynamic process of wrestling with the most challenging life events and parts of ourselves. "We will pass through them [these life issues] again and again, each time with a new story, each time with a greater understanding, until they become indistinguishable from our blessings and our wisdom. It's the way life teaches us how to live" (Remen 1996, xxvi).

In the third part of this book, we listen to sage advice from the field, learning about things that people find helpful to them in moving along this path. Chapter 9 describes the role of community in helping people move positively through hardships. Talking about their journey and the support of peers, family, and friends all played a role in people's positive growth. In chapter 10 we focus on the role that gratitude and compassion play in the positive transformation. Chapter 11 spotlights the impact of reflection, whether through time in nature, mindfulness, yoga, or meditation, on the positive growth that people experience. In chapter 12, we hear about the importance of doing something, whether helping others or making positive changes to a situation or system so that what happened to them won't happen to someone else. In chapter 13 we learn about the role of spirituality, forgiveness, and doing the right thing in how these people coped with difficulty.

The final chapter is about choice. One of the most inspiring aspects of these stories is the common element of choice. The people in these stories made choices each step of the way—choices that empowered them, choices that moved them along a positive path, wise choices that in the end made them better people and better doctors, and made the world a better place because they are a part of it. As one doctor put it, "I realized at some point that I had a choice. I could choose to stay in this dark place or I could choose to get out of it. And that made all the difference, knowing I had a choice." In the end, this book is about choosing wisdom.

2. Defining Wisdom

I want to beg you, as much as I can, to be patient toward all that is unsolved in your heart and to try to love the questions themselves like locked rooms and like books that are written in a very foreign tongue. Do not seek the answers, which cannot be given you because you would not be able to live them. And the point is to live everything. Live the questions now. Perhaps you will then gradually, without noticing it, live along some distant day into the answer. —RAINER MARIA RILKE

Wisdom is a love affair with questions. Knowledge is a love affair with answers. —JULIO OLALLA

IF THE EXPERIENCE of centuries of seekers is indicative, then we must acknowledge up front that, in spite of this chapter's title, we will not find answers to the question, "What is wisdom?" Simply asking the question and struggling with the idea, however, have the potential to help us become better people, so we learn to love the question, in all its complexity and nuance. Asking the question at the outset, with our eyes open, helps us to be better observers of the people we hear from in this volume. So we ask the question, not really expecting to come up with an answer, but knowing that the ideas we explore may resonate in the stories we hear, and then we might find the real meaning of wisdom for our own lives.

Wisdom is a vexing concept. We might think we know what it is, but when someone asks "What is wisdom?" most of us are left speechless for a moment, which we find both embarrassing and annoying. Once we regain our composure, we might say something like, "Well, I know it when I see it." There is indeed something to the notion that wisdom is difficult to describe, but we can identify it when we see it demonstrated. Wisdom has a multidimensional nature that words cannot fully capture; it is so integrated within action and context that it does not lend itself to a static definition. Although research on wisdom has been growing, no consensus has emerged on a definition. As one of the most prominent wisdom researchers noted, "Wisdom is about as elusive as psychological constructs get" (Sternberg 1990, ix). Common themes, though, run through the literature.

One approach is that wisdom is multidimensional, involving intellect as well as emotion, compassion, empathy, and self-reflection, and is embodied in the person (Ardelt 2004; Clayton 1982). Another viewpoint emphasizes wisdom as "expert knowledge, involving good judgment and advice in the (domain) fundamental pragmatics of life" (Baltes and Smith 1990). It is intimately connected with the conduct of life and with applying knowledge to right action and is often best recognized in the decisions we make in challenging life situations (Sternberg 2000). One feature of this expert knowledge, so well exemplified by Socrates and Job, is awareness of what we *don't* know, and understanding the extent to which life is uncertain (Baltes and Smith 1990; Sternberg 1990). This fundamental component of humility makes the study of wisdom particularly difficult, since, as wisdom researcher Monika Ardelt notes, wise persons are not likely to think or say that they are wise. The final theme is that, excluding those rare individuals such as the Buddha, it is not at all clear that any person ever has, or ever could, completely embody wisdom. But rather it is more likely that we ordinary, or even extraordinary, humans embody wisdom in some ways, at some times, or in some facets of our lives, and that growing wiser is more of a journey than a destination. While some people's lives exemplify wisdom more than others', perhaps all of us have exemplary moments when our thoughts or actions embody qualities of wisdom. In that way each choice and each action become opportunities. In the end, wisdom implies integration of knowledge, experience, humility, and compassion into a creative, good life—a life that makes the world a better place.

WISDOM THROUGHOUT HISTORY

The notion of wisdom has a rich history, with religious, philosophical, psychological, sociological, and most recently, neurobiological attempts to capture its essence. As we try to develop a conscious understanding of what wisdom is in terms of our own lives, let's get some help from history. One word of caution: As you dive into thinking about wisdom, you will no doubt get excited and inspired just thinking about it. You may find that you begin to ask yourself, on a regular basis, *Was that wise—what I just did?* This issue will then grow even more complex, as you begin to reflect on more general attributes: *Am I compassionate?* or *How do I deal with uncertainty?* or *Am I able to see things from many perspectives?* You will likely want to read more, and I refer you to the references section of this book.

Socrates

Our helicopter tour of the wisdom landscape begins with the philosophical tradition. When we think of wise people, one who often comes to mind is the great thinker and teacher Socrates. Socrates is known to us through the writings of his student, Plato, who recorded his teachings as well as his trial for impiety and corrupting the young (Plato 1950). As Plato chronicles, Socrates had been accused of "criminal meddling, in that he *inquires* into things below the earth and in the sky and makes the weaker argument defeat the stronger, and teaches others to follow his example" (*Apology* 17A, 17D–19D). The Oracle at Delphi had declared that "None is more wise than Socrates," but Socrates himself (with the humility characteristic of wise people) rejected that notion and set out to find others who might be wiser than he. That's where the trouble began.

Recall Julio Olalla's statement, "Wisdom is a love affair with questions, knowledge is a love affair with answers." Socrates perhaps best represents the primacy of questions in the quest for wisdom. As Stephen Hall expresses it so beautifully, "Socrates wielded his questions like a box cutter" (Hall 2010, 21), challenging both the questioner and the questioned, inquiring particularly into the extent to which we know things. Through his questions, he ruthlessly exposed the fact that our knowing is limited. In doing so, he gave us one of the most fundamental constructs of wisdom: humility.

According to Socrates the one who is continually aware of what he does not know is the wiser. "The wisest of you men is he who has realized, like Socrates, that in respect of wisdom he is really worthless" (Plato, *Apology* 22E–24A). Through Plato's writings we also begin to see the idea of the Good, and the notion that wisdom follows from understanding the Good. The idea then emerges that wisdom is understanding the deeper meaning of things. The Greek philosophers recognized that wisdom could be conceptualized as *phronesis*, or practical wisdom, and *sophia*, or the pursuit of timeless and universal truths through contemplation (Robinson 1990, 13–24). In Aristotle's writings we have a clear notion that wisdom is not just about what you know, but how you apply that knowledge in making good decisions. Furthermore, wisdom is signified by a life lived in accordance with *aretis*, or excellence (Aristotle, *Metaphysics* 1.1).

Thus, very early human thought noted that wisdom has many dimensions, involves humility, and has to do not only with thinking but how one lived.

Job

Stories from spiritual traditions offer some of these same themes. In the Judeo-Christian tradition, the story of Job is a stunning example of humility and another characteristic of wise persons: the ability to tolerate ambiguity. The book of Job teems with questions; most remain unanswered, but that might be the whole point. Job is surrounded by friends who think they know all about life and why Job is suffering. They are all full of advice. Job's wisdom is in his clear-eyed view of reality—his acceptance of the ambiguity implicit in the fact that he is a good person and he is also suffering. He rejects the more simplistic, judgmental, dichotomous view of the world, and in doing so begins to see the bigger picture, a more complex and less human-centric view of God and Creation. Perhaps most important, Job gives us a sense that wisdom is not so much about answers as it is about questions, and about the continuous struggle to discern the deeper meaning of things and to act in accordance with that discernment.

Buddha

In an amazing story of transformation from the East, Siddhartha Gautama set out on a journey to enlightenment (Strong 2001; Cantwell 2010). The journey began when the young prince, brought up in a life of privilege, was awakened to the universal experience of aging, suffering, and death. As the story is told, he renounced his former life and set out on a journey to "renounce the worldly life and work single mindedly for the appeasement of birth and death and the resultant attainment of peace and enlightenment" (Cantwell 30). The Buddha (to be) sought out two extraordinary meditation teachers and mastered their meditation systems, but "remained dissatisfied, since neither attainment brought liberation from the sorrows of life, so in each case he moved on" (32). He then immersed himself in the austerities, self-imposed disciplines "taken to their limit, such that no aesthetic could take them farther" (33). His body deteriorated, wasted away almost to the point of death. He finally concluded that such severe physical punishment "has no benefit, and is in fact detrimental to real spiritual progress, making the body too weak to meditate effectively. Thus, he began to eat again, and this provided strength for the meditations which led to his awakening" (33). An important point here is that the life of the Buddha points to a "Middle Way" between self-indulgence and extreme self-denial. The story also leaves open the question whether the enlightenment that the Buddha eventually achieves was only possible because of these years of suffering.

What happens next is the extraordinary story of the enlightenment and takes place under a bodhi tree. First, the Buddha (to be) is challenged by Mara, "the Buddhist devil symbolizing ignorance and attachment" (34), and an epic struggle ensues. With the help of the Earth as his witness, "Mara's legions are scattered in disarray" and the Buddha enters his final meditations to enlightenment. The enlightenment takes place later that night—specifically during the three watches of the night—when the Buddha acquires what are called the three knowledges. In the first watch of the night, the Buddha reviews all of his former lives, all of his births and deaths, and this review "shows the process of enlightenment to be the result of ongoing and continuous striving of one karmic individual" but also demonstrates that this karmic individual has no single self and is many different beings reborn with many different identities (Strong 2001, 74). In the second watch of the night, the Buddha turns his mind toward the other, and recognizes that there is no place of refuge from death and rebirth, and that the laws of karma apply to all beings, demonstrating the compassion of Buddha. In the third watch, the Buddha turns his mind toward the realization of "reality as it is," and this is often paired with the realization of the "Four Noble Truths: the truth of suffering, of the origin of suffering, of the cessation of suffering and of the path to the cessation of suffering" (Strong 2001, 75). As related by Strong, these four truths were the subject of the Buddha's first sermon in the deer park and became a fundamental tenant of the Buddhist tradition.

In the months that follow, Buddha begins to teach and through teaching about the Middle Way and the Four Noble Truths, goes on to give a road map of sorts, a lifelong process toward awakening (the Eightfold Path) that can end people's suffering. This path includes right view, right intention, right speech, right action, right livelihood, right effort, right mindfulness, and right concentration. Through this Eightfold Path, one comes to experience an enlightened view of reality in which there is no separate self. What Buddha is describing is a way of being in the world that reduces, and can eliminate, suffering. Compassion, interconnectedness, a continuous path of discernment, mindfulness, the capacity to overcome (or let go of) individual desires—these are all themes in this amazing story that we hear echoed in our modern understanding of wisdom.

Contemporary Thinkers: Wisdom and Psychology

Not until the early 1980s did modern science take up the notion of wisdom. As you can imagine, wisdom was a messy topic for science—

full of ambiguity, peppered with spiritual notions, layered with the annoying component of humility that made it even more difficult to study directly. Erik Erikson had opened the door to the psychological consideration of wisdom in referring to wisdom as the eighth and final stage of human development, but V. P. Clayton and J. E. Birren (1980) conceived some of the first scientific studies examining the nature of wisdom, starting with investigating common notions about it. They found that respondents considered wisdom "an attribute representing the integration of general cognitive, affective and reflective qualities" (118); in other words, wisdom was complex and multidimensional, involving emotion and the intellect.

Since then, numerous studies have documented this multidimensional nature of wisdom. P. B. Baltes and colleagues took on the task of applying rigorous scientific methodology to the study of the very complex concept of wisdom. They did so with complete awareness of the difficulties and potential limitations. They approached wisdom with the desire to understand the highest level of human performance and successful aging, and chose to study wisdom as manifested in how people respond to life dilemmas. Baltes and Smith define wisdom as "expert knowledge involving good judgment and advice in the domain, fundamental pragmatics of life (i.e., the important matters of life)" (Baltes and Smith 1990, 95). They further defined this expert knowledge system by developing explicit criteria by which they could then measure wisdom in an experimental context, giving study participants hypothetical life problem scenarios and evaluating their responses based on these criteria. For Baltes and the Berlin group, wisdom involved knowledge about important and difficult matters in life, knowledge about uncertainty and the limits of knowing, knowledge about differences in values and goals, and an understanding of context. Wisdom was best measured by contemplating hypothetical real-life dilemmas. So Baltes and his Berlin group defined wisdom in the context of action, as it related to the conduct of life.

R. J. Sternberg is another influential contemporary wisdom researcher whose work helps us to understand the differences between wisdom and intelligence and gives some insight into why being really smart doesn't necessarily get you a spot on the list of wise people. In an earlier study, Sternberg explored people's implicit theories of wisdom as they were differentiated from creativity and intelligence. He asked college students and professors to list and then sort behaviors that they felt characterized wisdom, as opposed to intelligence and creativity. For wisdom, six components emerged:

1. Reasoning ability
2. Sagacity (concern for others, self-knowledge, the ability to learn from mistakes)
3. Learning from ideas and the environment (being perceptive and learning from others' mistakes)
4. Good judgment
5. Expeditious use of information
6. Perspicacity (having intuition, recognizing right and truth, seeing through things, reading between the lines)

According to Sternberg, wisdom resists automatic thinking and seeks to understand wisdom in others. Wisdom seeks understanding of the deeper meaning of things as well as the limits of knowledge and understanding. Wisdom tolerates and seeks to understand ambiguity better, whereas intelligence seeks to eliminate ambiguity. Wisdom seeks to grasp what is known and what it means; intelligence, on the other hand, pursues knowledge and uses what is known, and creativity seeks to go beyond what is known (Sternberg 1990). Contrasting the three constructs of wisdom, intelligence, and creativity is useful, since there is overlap, but we do intuitively know the difference, and the contrast helps us to understand wisdom more clearly. The qualities that Sternberg attributes to wisdom are apparent in Socrates, who resisted the automatic thinking of his day, challenged others to see the limits of what they knew, and put on the table the ambiguous nature of reality. But how does a wise person actually make decisions when faced with complex life events? What guides him or her in navigating the often conflicting set of values? In more recent work, Sternberg has developed what he terms the "Balance Theory" of wisdom. Here, he conceptualizes wisdom as "the application of intelligence and experience as mediated by values toward the achievement of a *common good* through a balance among (1) intrapersonal, (2) interpersonal, and (3) extrapersonal interests, over the (1) short and (2) long terms, to achieve a balance among (1) adaptation to existing environments, (2) shaping of existing environments, and (3) selection of new environments (Sternberg 2004, 165). This sounds complicated, but it gives you a sense of the complexity of making wise decisions and the importance of self-reflection and the ability to transcend ourselves when facing life's most challenging situations. It also brings front and center the *common good* as the ultimate value guiding the decisions of wise persons.

Fast-forward to another pioneering researcher in the field of wisdom studies, Monika Ardelt. Building on work by Clayton and Birren, and bringing back the multidimensional focus, Ardelt has focused her work on wise persons. In a review of how psychologists have operationalized wisdom, Ardelt argues for the wholeness of wisdom, that "the definition, operationalization and measurement of wisdom should not be reduced to expertise and . . . the term wisdom should be reserved for wise persons rather than expert knowledge" (Ardelt 2004, 257). She advocates for wisdom being studied with attention to how wise persons are, rather than simply assessing their expert or intellectual knowledge. Ardelt further develops the three-dimensional construct of wisdom, made up of cognitive, affective, and reflective components. The *cognitive* component is described as an understanding of life and a desire to know the truth, i.e., to comprehend the significance and deeper meaning of phenomena and events, particularly with regard to intrapersonal and interpersonal matters. [This] includes knowledge and acceptance of the positive and negative aspects of human nature, of the inherent limits of knowledge, and of life's unpredictability and uncertainties" (275). The *affective* dimension of wisdom manifests as sympathetic and compassionate love for others, which increase as self-centeredness is transcended (recall the story of Buddha). The *reflective* component of wisdom represents "self-examination, self-awareness, self-insight and the ability to look at phenomena and events from different perspectives"

(Ardelt 2004, 275). This reflective component is seen as something that promotes the further development of wisdom, because it allows people to reflect on their experience—to learn, change, and grow wiser. Reflection also protects us from becoming entrenched in a particular stance, as it promotes our consideration of things from different perspectives and helps us to be aware of our own fears, biases, and projections.

Common Themes

At this point you might be feeling a little overwhelmed by all the different ways in which wisdom has been conceptualized. But when we scan the landscape from spiritual, philosophical, and psychological perspectives, it's striking how many more similarities there are than differences, and the common themes begin to coalesce into a coherent concept.

To summarize, completely wise people might appear something like this: They understand the deeper meaning of things, resist automatic thinking, and are able to see things from many perspectives. They understand and can tolerate the ambiguity in life; they desire to know the truth and can see through simplistic, black-and-white thinking that hides the ambiguous truth. They are aware of and can acknowledge the limits of what they know. They are compassionate and capable of seeing things from the perspective of others. They have a clear-eyed view of reality and can see things as they are. They are humble and able to acknowledge and learn from mistakes, both their own and others'. They are concerned with the deeper meaning of things, always seeking to understand, which is why they are in love with questions.

How can we begin to understand more about wisdom?

Job Revisited

If what Baltes says is true, and wisdom is something that we can recognize when we see it in action (1990, 107), then perhaps the best way to learn more about wisdom is to observe and to listen. Where do we go to find it? Do we look for those exemplary individuals who are wise on a grand scale, or can we find wisdom in ordinary people? I don't know about you, but the numbers of people I can name whom I would consider "ultimately wise" or "perfectly wise" are very few. Even those I would consider very wise have made plenty of bad decisions and lacked compassion at times; in other words, they're hardly perfectly wise. Plenty of people, though, manifest in big and small ways the characteristics of wisdom we've been talking about, and we can learn much from them.

Let's revisit Job as an example of wisdom in action. In the book named for him, the path to wisdom is found in Job's coping with and responding to suffering. The biblical wisdom literature stresses practical wisdom, related to questions about life rather than questions about knowing, about coping first and understanding later, because the understanding comes out of the coping. Job suffers every imaginable plague, pestilence, and pain, as well as the continuous advice and answers from his religious and righteous friends who think they have wisdom but who are, in the Socratic sense, truly ignorant. In trying to explain Job's suffering, they conjure up reasons to blame Job for his own suffering. But Job remains steadfast in his belief that he is a good man, that this suffering is something that he cannot understand: "Oh, that I had one to hear me! (Here is my signature! Let the Almighty answer me!) Oh, that I had the indictment written by my adversary!" (Job 31:35). Interestingly, Job never gets a straight answer from God, but he continues to wait and listen and believe, and somehow in the context of his experience, an answer becomes unnecessary. In his new relationship with God (new in his clear-eyed realization that just being good does not protect him from suffering), Job is able to accept the ambiguous nature of life. "I know that thou canst do all things, and that no purpose of thine can be thwarted. Who is this who hides counsel without knowledge: therefore I have uttered what I did not understand, things too wonderful for me, which I did not know. Hear, and I will speak: I will question you and you declare to me. I had heard of thee by the hearing of the ear, but now my eye sees thee" (Job 42:2–5). This intimate relationship with God, this new and clear vision (a view of the deeper meaning of things), and this deep humility came through Job's experience of suffering, and was a gift so amazing as to make vindication superfluous. Job became a living example of humility, knowing the limits of his knowledge and understanding of the deeper meaning in life. Sound familiar? Sounds like wisdom in action. The humbling thing about this story is that we are left wondering how Job did that. Appropriately, we are left with a question, and hopefully we are changed, just a little bit, by the experience of listening—really listening—to Job or others like Job who cope with difficulties and gain wisdom from their experience.

Wise Elders

Monika Ardelt studies wise elders. These are not famous people or monks who meditate eighteen hours a day. Ardelt has focused on identifying wisdom in ordinary people, particularly ordinary older people. In the Personality and Aging Well Study, Ardelt and her colleagues surveyed 180 older adults using her three-dimensional wisdom scale. She then followed up with in-depth interviews of those who scored highest and lowest on the scale to investigate how these individuals dealt with hardship and difficulties in life.

James was a seventy-seven-year-old African American retired school administrator. As Ardelt describes him in her wonderful article, "How Wise People Cope with Crisis and Obstacles in Life" (2005), James was a World War II veteran who "witnessed death and destruction, and slipped into a depression after he returned from the war and saw 'how reckless and carelessly Americans were living'" (10). Ardelt investigates how James and two other wise individuals had dealt with hardship in their lives. She notes, "All three had difficulties thinking about their most unpleasant events . . . because there was a general consensus that life is good and enjoyable" (11). Once she manages to elicit from them how they dealt with their hardships, she finds that wise elders appear to use three higher-order strategies. First, they "mentally distanced themselves from the situation by taking a step back to relax and calm down. Second, they actively coped with the challenge by doing whatever needed to be done and could be done and third, they applied the life lessons that they had learned" (11). James put it this way: "I've had as [many] bad things . . . happen as good things, but I've never allowed any outside force to take possession of my being. That means, whenever I had a problem, I went to something wholesome to solve it. . . . I did not pick up any outside things to solve my problems, like smoking or drinking. . . . And I think that if there would be more of that with young people now, we would get them learning how to solve their problems differently other than blaming someone else and taking it out in violent ways" (12). As Ardelt observes, James learned to deal with the uncertainties in life in part through his faith, but his faith was engaged through his actions and those of others. He describes it this way: "And you know the Almighty is in it, but it comes through people. It gives you all the confidence in the world in people. And things aren't going to be right all the time, but there's pleasant things to happen" (13).

James's approach contrasts with how the low-wisdom elders cope with hardship. First, they do not have difficulty thinking of troubling experiences; they use a passive coping strategy, including resignation to their circumstances, and a passive reliance on God to intervene on their behalf; and they do not engage in any self-reflective activities.

If we are listening, there are plenty of stories to hear. We find that when people have learned something the hard way, they naturally want to share that with others. In fact, the sharing of stories might not only help the listener, but it may also help the teller. In telling the story, the teller might actually gain more insight into her own experiences. By telling or writing the story, and sharing it with others, we are both discovering and sharing wisdom.

WISDOM AND THE ROLE OF STORIES

In many traditions, wisdom is shared through stories. Physician and author Rachel Naomi Remen writes in her excellent book, *Kitchen Table Wisdom* (1996), "Sitting around the table telling stories is not just a way of passing time. It is the way the wisdom gets passed along. This stuff that helps us to live a life worth remembering" (xxvii). She adds, "Despite the awesome power of technology, many of us still do not live very well. We may need to listen to each other's stories once again" (xxvii). She goes on to caution that "real stories take time," and that, in this fast-paced world, we often have to be stopped in our tracks by events unforeseen; only then do we, as she puts it, "take a seat at the kitchen table" (xxvii) to listen to others' stories of wisdom and to tell our own. In the telling and the listening, meaning is discovered and wisdom is shared: "We carry with us every story we have ever heard and every story we have ever lived, filed away at some deep place in our memory. We carry most of those stories unread, as it were, until we have grown the capacity or the readiness to read them. When that happens, they may come back to us filled with a previously unsuspected meaning. It is almost as if we have been collecting pieces of greater wisdom, sometimes over many years, without knowing" (xxxi). Stories are likely to be the best way to capture the way to wisdom, individually and collectively.

But before we become observers, we need to understand a few more concepts. This book is about wisdom emerging out of adversity. But why adversity? Can suffering lead to wisdom? Monika Ardelt thinks so. In fact, she says in the film *Choosing Wisdom*, "The fastest way to wisdom is through adversity in life." Judith Gluck and colleagues used narrative to study the development of wisdom (Gluck 2005). They asked people to write three different stories: one about a time when they acted wisely, one when they were foolish, and one about a "peak experience." They then analyzed the narratives and found that they differed significantly. The wisdom stories were about important and meaningful life events and, specifically, were more often about difficult or negative events than were the peak experience or foolish narratives, suggesting that perhaps negative events may be important in the formation of wisdom. Juan Pascual-Leone described adversity situations or what he calls "limit situations" as overwhelming, unavoidable, and apparently irresolvable

life events (Pascual-Leone 2000). He calls "ultimate limit situations:
ones that cannot be undone and are nonetheless faced with consciousness and resolve . . . situations like death, illness . . . absolute failure
. . . uncontrollable fear" (247). He suggests that confronting these situations with awareness and resolve can lead to remarkable growth in the
self and the natural emergence of the transcendent self—"if the situations do not destroy the person first" (247). What is it about adversity
that helps us develop wisdom? Lawrence Calhoun and his colleagues
have some clues in what they term "posttraumatic growth," which is
the subject of the next chapter.

3. Posttraumatic Growth

What doesn't kill me makes me stronger.
—FRIEDRICH NIETZSCHE

HOW CAN SUFFERING LEAD TO WISDOM?

BEFORE WE GET into ideas about how adversity can result in anything positive, let me say right up front that lots of bad things can happen as a result of adversity. That being said, adversity appears to be so universal as to be unavoidable at some point in our lives. Fortunately, not all of us will suffer catastrophic loss or pain, but we all endure some loss and pain. In fact, we frequently experience small obstacles, losses, or pain. What becomes of us in the aftermath of those experiences, big and small? What can we learn from each other about how to have the best chance of coming out of such experiences stronger, more compassionate, and yes, wiser? The experience of difficulty, whether major or minor, offers the possibility for change, for worse or for better. What about that experience makes it an opportunity for wisdom?

Let's think in general about the characteristics of wisdom that we heard about in the previous chapter, characteristics that emerge as themes throughout the centuries of people thinking about wisdom. One of the properties generally accepted as inherent in the definition of wisdom is understanding the limits of our knowledge. Wise people know that they can't know everything and are humble in the awareness of the limitations of their understanding. Another commonly accepted component of wisdom is the awareness that life circumstances are often ambiguous, and that life is uncertain and messy. A wise person can see and accept that and work with it. Also found in most descriptions of wisdom are the components of empathy, compassion, and the ability to transcend self-centeredness. All these elements imply the ability to accept the limitations as well as the potential in life circumstances and to continuously search for and create meaning in life's events.

Ask yourself: What kind of life experience might reawaken us to the uncertainty of life, remind us of the limits of what we know, help us connect with others who are suffering, and open us up to the possibility of change? Adversity presents the greatest of all challenges to what we know about ourselves and about the meaning of our lives. Empathy and compassion are borne of suffering. An unexpected and difficult turn of events reminds us of the uncertainty in life. Appreciation of the limits of knowledge likewise comes from our experience of things we cannot understand, and tolerance of ambiguity is likely borne of situations that we can neither understand nor control. So there we have it in a nutshell: adversity becomes one of our greatest teachers of wisdom.

We're not talking about just coping, or even resilience, which implies being able to bounce back. We're talking about coming out of a very difficult experience as a better and wiser person. This way of thinking about the human response to trauma is fairly new, pioneered by psychologists Lawrence Calhoun and Richard Tedeschi. They call it *posttraumatic growth*.

Can We Respond to Adversity in a Positive Way?

Posttraumatic growth, a psychological construct that emerged in the mid-1990s, refers to a positive psychological response in the wake of trauma that goes beyond the concept of resilience to a process of positive transformation. Tedeschi and Calhoun have worked with trauma patients for many years, and they noticed in their clinical practice that many years after the trauma, some people were able to look back and point out how the very difficult circumstance they experienced transformed them in a positive fashion. Prior to this, much of the work on trauma had been focused on negative effects. Calhoun and Tedeschi began interviewing trauma survivors and asking questions about what they learned and how they had changed in a positive way. Their research, along with the research of other pioneering colleagues in the field, has changed how we think about psychological trauma and can help us understand how we can help patients (and each other) not just to cope in the aftermath of trauma but to learn how we can grow.

Tedeschi and Calhoun describe the positive changes that can occur in the wake of severe trauma as a complex, positive, transformational response that falls into five domains:

1. Greater appreciation for life and changed sense of priorities
2. Warmer, more intimate relationships with others
3. Recognition of new possibilities or paths for one's life
4. Greater sense of personal strength
5. Spiritual development

In the process of this positive transformation, people go beyond coping and are able to step forward in their development—toward what looks a lot like wisdom. Tedeschi and Calhoun developed a framework of how this posttraumatic growth takes place (see Figure 1).

Tedeschi and Calhoun posit that people facing adversity move through a process of rumination and, with the help of self-disclosure and engaging social support, are able to reconfigure their self-understanding/understanding of the world (their *schema*), rework their life story, and emerge with positive growth.

Researcher Ronnie Janoff-Bulman characterizes three different ways that trauma survivors might experience positive changes. First, they often discover newfound personal strength in the aftermath of a difficult event. Second, they may undergo an existential reevaluation (wrestling with the question of why evil exists in the world); in the process, they may come to accept ambiguity and the fragile nature of life, and gain a greater appreciation for life itself and the ordinary things we take for granted. They may also develop a greater appreciation for the things they do have control over and the choices they make, and they may restructure how they spend their time or be more intentional about their choices. Finally, survivors may be more psychologically prepared for future events. Besides recalling their increased strength, they may

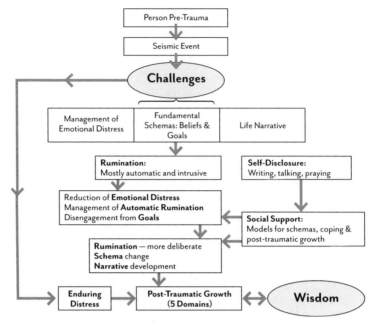

FIGURE 1. A MODEL OF POSTTRAUMATIC GROWTH

Richard Tedeschi and Lawrence Calhoun (2004). "Posttraumatic Growth:
Conceptual Foundations and Empirical Evidence." *Psychological Inquiry* 15(1): 7.

also develop a view of the world that can assimilate difficulties and
challenges, much like a building that has been fitted to bend and sway
with an earthquake.

The Process of Coping

We can benefit from understanding what Tedeschi and Calhoun have
identified as some of the key cognitive processing activities that people
engage in when coping with traumatic experiences. It is important to
note that the type of event is perhaps not the major determinant of how
traumatic the event feels. Janoff-Bulman points out that "it is not the
recognizable . . . external losses . . . that define the event as traumatic,
but rather the internal disorganization and disintegration that follows
from our psychological unpreparedness" (2006, 83). Our discussion,
then, focuses on the *process* of coping rather than the event itself, recog-

nizing that the same event experienced by different people in different circumstances may have very different effects.

The most difficult events are those that challenge what psychologists call our *schemas*—our most fundamental assumptions about the world. In the story of Job, the fundamental understanding that was being challenged was the idea that good works and good people are rewarded; at least they aren't punished. This schema was so deeply embedded in the religious assumptions of Job's day that his story represents a radical departure from the norm. The people around Job are clearly stuck in this schema, coming to the conclusion that Job must have done something to deserve his situation. The parallels to our modern desire to assign fault and blame are all too obvious in our current judgmental world. We search for reasons to blame rather than acknowledging the ambiguity of life. Job's friends were just like that, and their foolishness stemmed from their inability to see reality in all its messiness and to allow their rigid schemas to be challenged. Job's wisdom was found in his capacity to realize that he was a good, faithful person *and* he was also suffering. The two could coexist. While he didn't understand what brought his bad fortune, he would continue to listen and reflect. Eventually, he lived his way into a more expanded understanding of God and his own place in the world—one that was less human-centric, less rigid, and more tolerant of ambiguity.

Rumination

Just as a bicycle's wheels are essential for its progress, a key cognitive process involved in posttraumatic growth is *rumination*. Rumination has a fairly negative connotation. Perhaps someone has said to you exasperatedly, "Stop ruminating and go *do* something." Plenty of evidence supports the idea that *negative* rumination can be destructive, and *persistent negative* rumination (intrusive thoughts about a traumatic event) is part of the diagnostic criteria for posttraumatic stress disorder. But rumination is not all bad. In fact, it appears to be solidly associated with posttraumatic growth (Calhoun and Tedeschi 2000; Janoff-Bulman 2006). Rachel Naomi Remen wrote, "We carry with us every story we have ever heard and every story we have ever lived. . . . It is almost as if we have been collecting pieces of a greater wisdom, sometimes over many years without knowing" (1996, xxxi). At any point, with positive rumination, those stories can come back to us with new meaning.

Rumination involves going over the negative event, a feeling that one must discuss the event, and a search for meaning (Tait and Silver 1989). As we'll see, all these actions are important to moving through trauma; therefore, rumination can be like the wheel of a bike, slowly moving us through important steps toward the goal of recovery. The wheel may get stuck, however, and rumination may increase when goals of recovery are not met (Martin and Tesser 1996, 16). Calhoun and Tedeschi make a distinction between an early form of intrusive rumination that may be useful in helping us slowly take in the reality of what has happened (moving through denial at our own pace) and to seek out help (moving toward disclosure) and a later, more deliberate and reflective form of rumination (Calhoun and Tedeschi 2006). This later, more deliberate and reflective form of rumination serves to repair, or restructure and rebuild our understanding of ourselves and the world (Janoff-Bulman 2006; Clark 1996).

Making Sense of the Event

A second important element in the process of posttraumatic growth involves *making sense of the event*. The opportunity for growth through adversity comes at least in part because our previous understanding of the world and ourselves is challenged or destroyed. The goal therefore becomes rebuilding that understanding in a way that encompasses the reality of what has happened. Essential to this rebuilding appears to be a process of making sense of the event, fitting it into a reconfigured understanding of the world. For the doctors in our study, the reality of having made a mistake that harmed a patient challenged to the core their previous schema that "good doctors don't make mistakes." With that understanding and the current reality, the only available courses of action seemed to be quitting medicine or, in the worst-case scenario, committing suicide, which certainly happens in the wake of medical mistakes. In order to go on living, some adjustment must be made to the prior understanding of the world and this doctor's place in it—one that allows the physician to be vulnerable to mistakes, just as other humans are.

With rumination as a tool, how do we go about the process of taking in a shattering event and allowing it to shape a new understanding of ourselves and the world? One key piece of the puzzle seems to be finding meaning in what happened. Researcher Mel Lerner (2010) noted that humans need to be able to make sense of what has happened, even if it means finding fault inappropriately (think about Job's "friends"). If we do not allow the situation to shatter our former worldview, we strive to fit the current reality into the former schema, like putting a square peg into a round hole. If you pound hard enough, you can actually get it in (sometimes), but you destroy a lot of wood along the way and it never really fits.

Those with a perfectionist mind-set might make a mistake, and rather than allowing that mistake to challenge understanding of themselves as capable of perfection, they say to themselves, *Well, if I just try harder, and I'm more vigilant, I can, in fact, be perfect.* This attitude is fairly common in medicine. Unfortunately and inevitably, the doctor—a few days or years later—makes another mistake. Failing to revise our understanding of ourselves prevents us from seeing our reality. In medicine, that means preventing us from taking the truly helpful steps of creating systems around us that acknowledge our human imperfection.

The drive to make sense of things can, on the other hand, lead to growth and expansion or a positive revision of our understanding of ourselves and the world. But the way through takes courage, and perhaps some optimism; the way from incomprehensibility to sensemaking requires a time of chaos, which can be terrifying—being in the rubble and realizing that the schema we had is truly destroyed and no longer real.

C. S. Lewis was one of the most esteemed theologians of his time. But in the aftermath of his wife's untimely death at the age of fifty, Lewis likened his faith to a house of cards, not the solid and unshakable faith that he thought it was. If one's faith is built on a fundamental belief that God has a purpose, then suffering and untimely death present fundamental challenges to the concept of a God who is good and just. In the face of that challenge, many find their faith shaken. What they thought they understood—about God, about the world—now makes no sense. The world these traumatized people knew is no more, and there is no way around it. They are left to pick their way through the rubble of their former worldview and the reality of their current life, trying to find a way to put it all together. How do we pick up the pieces?

Integration

Janoff-Bulman suggests that this recognition of the meaninglessness of existence is the beginning of a new sense of meaning and value. As she describes it, survivors begin to incorporate the fact that human fragility and vulnerability are realities that cannot be ignored, and that, over time, these initially threatening realities "cease to wholly define the survivor's inner world" (Janoff-Bulman 2006, 89). "They become integrated into a set of assumptions that are now less absolutist and presumably more complex. They do not disappear, but are a part of a larger assumptive world that increasingly recognizes that the world is benevolent, but not always, and the world is comprehensible, but not always" (89). So begins the possibility of meaning-making.

A shift occurs right about here, in which what we had previously taken for granted is now appreciated and valued in an entirely different way. C. S. Lewis, after a long and tumultuous struggle with his own faith, wrote toward the end of his diary *A Grief Observed*, "We cannot understand. The best is perhaps what we understand the least" (1961, 89). The recognition of the reality of insecurity and the frailty of human life is followed by an enhanced appreciation of that which *is* at the current moment. This greater awareness of and appreciation for life can lead to living a better life, a life more cognizant of the important things, more intentional, more aware, and wiser. This change in our understanding of ourselves and our place in the world, and eventually in the way that we live our lives, becomes the meaning that we derive from difficult circumstances.

As we noted in chapter 2, one way that people seem to be able to discover meaning in their experience and therefore grow, is in the writing or the telling of our "stories." Physician and teacher of medicine Rita Charon puts it this way, "By telling stories to ourselves and others . . . in dreams, in diaries, in friendships, in marriages, in therapy sessions . . . we grow slowly not only to know who we are but to become who we are" (2006, vii). In other words, the telling of the story changes us. James Pennebaker did an interesting study in which he had people write for fifteen minutes on four consecutive days about a topic. The experimental group was asked to write about a traumatic experience, describing their deepest thoughts and feelings. The control group was asked to write about nonemotional topics. He then followed their overall health by recording their illness visits to the doctor over the subsequent year. What he found was extraordinary. Those who had written about their thoughts and feelings significantly reduced their doctor visits compared to the groups that wrote about trivial topics. In subsequent analyses of the narratives he demonstrated that those who did best were those whose narratives reflected discovery of meaning and insight into their circumstance (1999, 1249).

Finding Meaning

In many cases, finding meaning means actually doing something that *gives* meaning to the event. A traumatic event may be a catalyst to significant changes in the way people do things or in what they do, and those changes give meaning to the tragedy they have experienced. Many outstanding organizations that are catalysts for change were borne of adversity. Mothers Against Drunk Driving (MADD) was founded by mothers of children who were victims of drunk-driving incidents. Unspeakable grief gave birth to powerful change agents that moved not only individuals but an entire culture toward a better way. The family of James Brady (shot and permanently disabled during the assassination attempt on Ronald Reagan), families of the Virginia Tech shootings in 2007, and countless others have been moved by their tragedies to make sense of the loss through actions of mercy, compassion, and reason.

Many of the physicians in our study changed their career path to dedicate time and energy to improving patient safety. Others, like Dr. Jamie Redgrave in the film *Choosing Wisdom* that accompanies this volume, chose to spend more time with each patient, despite growing pressures to reduce patient visit time. Some patients began volunteering to help others in need, and some changed their careers to become therapists focused on helping pain patients. These changes were a large part of the meaning that they found in their own experience of suffering. All these people, in how they chose to respond, created meaning for their experience and in the process helped to improve the world. As a result, we progress not just as individuals but as a whole community.

The work of Calhoun and Tedeschi makes the point that, not only does individual positive transformation occur in the wake of trauma, but as the story of trauma is disclosed, support is shared and the reworking of the schema occurs collectively, so an entire community can share in the growth that occurs. The community is involved in collective reflection of the event's meaning, and the collective schema is potentially changed for the better. A collective awareness of the fragility of life can lead to a collective appreciation for life in the moment, a collective restructuring of priorities, and a collective expression of compassion and mercy. Some of our greatest moments as human beings and as societies came in the wake of suffering. In the United States, the New Deal was borne of the Great Depression, with a keen awareness of the suffering of hunger and poverty that struck people we knew to be good. Collectively, we vowed as a society to never again let our citizens suffer in that way, and the safety net of social security was born. Our society became more compassionate in the wake of the Depression, which had caused such widespread and undeniable suffering.

The collective experience of trauma, if processed collectively, can thus lead to collective, even societal, positive transformation. As we move further away from a trauma, however, we risk what Richard Bell calls "going to sleep" in relation to the lessons learned through suffering (Bell 2007, 1). The keen cultural awareness of the possibility of widespread hunger and poverty that afflicted not just a slice of our society but everyone is in our distant past. That distance makes us dangerously ignorant of the possibility of suffering in our own time in ways that defy our sense of righteousness and allows us to slip into a collective denial that this suffering might affect us, despite our good nature and high social stature.

Positive transformation does not mean, however, that the pain or difficulty disappears. As Janoff-Bulman puts it, trauma has a dual legacy. "It is important to realize that the benefits associated with trauma are inextricably tied to the pain and losses" (94). She makes the point that posttraumatic growth, like wisdom, includes recognition of the good and the bad, the positive and the negative. "[Survivors'] palpable awareness of vulnerability and loss, coupled with their rebuilt, generally positive assumptive world creates the climate for meaning, value, and commitment" (95).

At least for some people, adversity can apparently be a positive, transformational experience of growth. This positive transformation looks a lot like wisdom. In addition, the meaning found through suffering seems to lead to growth. We would also suggest that we develop wisdom and discover or create meaning in the process of responding to suffering.

We have established that wisdom is complex, multidimensional, and difficult to define, but that we know it when we see it. We have seen that adversity can be a double-edged sword, piercing the center of our being and causing great suffering but also opening up the possibility for growth and wisdom. How can we best prepare ourselves for the task ahead? Assuming that we would rather learn and grow as much as possible without having to suffer through what others do, what can we learn from each other? Maybe we can learn about wisdom from observing each other—particularly from those who have faced adversity.

A Theologian's Experience

Let's look a bit more closely at the experience of C. S. Lewis. He became his own observer in the aftermath of his wife's death, and he wrote it all down in *A Grief Observed* (1961). Lewis was a learned and religious man, well versed in Christian teachings and one of the most respected scholars of his day. When his wife died, he was stunned by the degree to which his suffering challenged his understanding of God, and in his grief he found solace and meaning by writing down his thoughts and feelings. He writes with the curiosity of someone outside himself, but with an intensity that comes from within. "No one ever told me that grief feels so much like fear," he states. "I'm not afraid, but the sensation is like being afraid . . . the same fluttering in the stomach, the same restlessness, the yawning" (1). Lewis is an astute observer of his experience of grief, including the challenges to his understanding of God, himself, and his place in the world. As readers we have the unusual opportunity to observe with him the aftermath of trauma and the process of moving through it. "When reality smashes my dream to bits, I mope and snarl while the first shock lasts, and then patiently, idiotically, start putting it together again? And so always? However often the house of cards falls, shall I set about rebuilding it? Is that what I am doing now?" (44). With ruthlessly honest self-reflection, Lewis then examines his faith and his life over time, slowly arriving at a new understanding that encompasses what cannot be understood. Most instructive in Lewis's account is his raw and unapologetic rendering of his situation, and his stance of nonjudgmental curiosity about his response. We are ultimately left with questions, but we have learned so much about his process and are grateful for the self-reflective window into his growth.

We can be observers, too—astute, quiet, nonjudgmental observers of those who have struggled with adversity. We ask questions and listen. We look for patterns. Most of all, we stand in awe and respect of the courage, strength, and wisdom that these trailblazing human beings exemplify. As astute observers, we might be able to learn something important, even lifesaving, by paying attention to their path. As the philosopher Søren Kierkegaard suggests, "Just by observing such a sufferer, one comes to know unmistakably what the highest is" (1938, 160).

PART TWO

The Path through Adversity

It's one step forward, one step back and then a step to the side. One day we are talking about growth, the next day I am in a deep dark hole and that growth stuff seems like a pile of crap to me.
—LAWRENCE CALHOUN, from the film *Choosing Wisdom*

Every step of the journey is the journey. —ZEN PROVERB

In part 2 we note that people take journeys through difficult circumstances to a place of greater wisdom. A journey implies some kind of path, but suggesting that this path is the same for everyone would be inaccurate. In fact, each person's journey is different, although some common elements promote our understanding of the process that people go through to cope positively with adversity. Not everyone's journey contains these elements, and in some people's experience one element is more important than another. Our intent is simply to give voice to what these exemplars describe in the hope that it will resonate with what others might experience. As you read, ask yourself how the stories and conclusions resonate with your own experiences of adversity and your own journey through trying times.

4. Acceptance

Acceptance of what has happened is the first step to overcoming the consequences of any misfortune. —William James

The curious paradox is that when I accept myself just as I am, then I can change. —Carl Rogers

Accepting a difficult life challenge often involves a change in direction. Instead of turning away from adversity we are turning toward it, approaching instead of avoiding. This shift in attitude leads to many new possibilities and begins with a welcome release from suffering and distress. Two stories of acceptance appear in this chapter—one of a physician and one of a patient with chronic pain. Their stories show that moving into acceptance can take time and is nourished in many ways; openness to new experience, support from others, developing nonjudgmental awareness, the motivation to have a meaningful life, letting go of negative feelings, and facing our human mortality and limitations all help turn the tide from suffering to growth. In both sets of stories, a burden is lifted and the narrative begins to shift. To set the stage for acceptance, let's first look at what precedes it: the emotional distress or suffering, the burden that is eventually eased.

Emotional Numbness

In the wake of a tragic life circumstance, there is often a phase of feeling overwhelmed or being in a state of not feeling at all—an emotional numbness in reaction to the shock. A natural response is to escape temporarily by diverting attention to something else or simply denying that the problem exists: *This just can't be happening to me.* Psychological theories of defending against or avoiding painful experience rest on the idea that sometimes life can be too overwhelming to experience all at once.

The gamut of negative emotions typically follows this initial phase. People vary in how they cope with trauma in the short term, depending on the situation, their personalities, and their personal history. Some people run away for a respite; others get angry and lash out by blaming someone else for the problem; still others fall apart under the weight of anxiety and guilt. The duration of this phase varies considerably from person to person and can last for years, especially without the positive support usually needed to emerge from the turmoil and come to terms with what has happened. The posttraumatic growth model explored in chapter 3 shows the shift from initially managing emotional distress to reducing it. At this point we begin to see growth. Overall, this phase is summarized in the model as enduring distress.

Dr. H is a pediatric surgeon who lived through one of life's most tragic circumstances—making a medical error that resulted in a patient's death. He found the first couple of days afterward overwhelming. As in other circumstances that involve sudden and unexpected death, the reality may simply be too much to comprehend immediately. In the documentary *Choosing Wisdom,* Lawrence Calhoun uses the metaphor of the aftermath of an earthquake to describe the emotional devastation left in the wake of a fatal medical mistake. People look dazed and grief-stricken, often standing motionless and seeming unable to process fully what has just happened. After making a critical medical error, physicians sometimes describe their immediate reactions as numbness, confusion, emotional distress, and the natural impulse to get some respite from it. In Dr. H's words,

> I think that time allows you not to think about things. I mean the next day I couldn't work, and part of it was I wanted that bad thing to go away, and I think I pushed it back so it wasn't so raw. I wanted

it to be very private. I didn't want other people to know that I had made a mistake.

Well, the whole time that this was going on, the lawsuit was happening and I couldn't sleep. I would wake up at night. I would sit up at night and my heart was pounding. I was beside myself with anxiety, fear, guilt. I felt terrible. For days, it was just turmoil—very distracted by the fact that someone had died on my watch, probably for a reason that was preventable.

You go through the looking glass. It's just a very bizarre world.

THE STORY OF DR. H:
"ALL I CAN THINK OF IS HIS NAME"

Dr. H tells his story of assisting in the surgery of a two-year-old boy when the boy suddenly died during what was supposed to be a relatively routine heart-valve repair.

My role in this resuscitation included multiple units of blood and cracking open his chest—I mean the whole nine yards—his not surviving and hearing the attending tell the family and hearing them fall apart. It was the most horrible nightmare I could imagine. This little boy had gone from somebody who maybe needed this repair and maybe didn't—he was asymptomatic—to dead.

The rest of the month I felt like I was just getting by. Somebody bumped into me in the hall and said, "Hi, how are you doing?" and I just started crying. I mean, I couldn't stop. I think everything had been bottled up. I couldn't even walk, so they sent me home.

At the end of his interview, Dr. H has an insight about a nightmare that he now interprets as trying to get him to deal with and accept the situation.

I did have a very weird dream between the day the boy died and my crying jag. I woke up suddenly. I had had a dream where this angel was saying, "You need to wake up," and I took her and I just shook her. I shook her really hard—and I woke up doing that. That was sort of my body, or God, saying, "You need to deal with this." But I did not wake up and say, "Oh, I need to deal with this." For the next eight years I would have flashbacks, and I would just be driving down the highway and think about it, or I'd conjure up horrible images. It was like a war scene, so bloody and gross. I could see his heart dying, and it was just horrible.

Then I had the opportunity to participate in a workshop where we were supposed to share a story of loss, and when I shared this story I fell apart. It was a way of being listened to, and after that I could feel this burden lifted off me. I stopped having those flashbacks, so it was a very powerful healing thing, but obviously it never goes away.

It doesn't just apply to medical situations. If you have the rug pulled out from under you, when things are just spiraling out of control and you can't do anything about it, that sense is universal, even though the circumstance may be different.

I am not afraid to keep asking people who have gone through a similar experience how they are doing. There were times when I could talk about it and other times when I couldn't. So I give them space and respect that, knowing how healing that can be.

I have faith that whatever happens I can get through this. I will be able to figure out what the meaning of all this is, that this is a test or a trial or a path that I have to walk at this moment. It may not make sense to me now, but it's going to be okay. You can get through the most horrible things. So having walked through that and being able to get to the other side of it is empowering.

The empathy factor is very big. I feel that instead of shying away from things like that, I feel I can be here through this. You can heal even if it seems like you can't when it happens. I want to be able to just let others know that it happens to the best of us and it's really hard, but it's a path and you aren't going to feel instantly better, but there are ways to feel better. I don't know how that is going to play out, but yeah, I do feel a desire to help people and give back.

I love interacting with families, and if there is some bad news or something to tell them, then I want someone like me to be the one to tell them. I don't want somebody at that moment in their lives to ever feel brushed off. I feel that it's very important, and I love working with those families and conveying that to the students and residents.

In Dr. H's story we see the progression from overwhelming trauma to acceptance. Years later, he has faith that people get through the most horrible things. Instead of shying away from difficult circumstances, he empathically strives to be a sensitive listener to others in distress.

THE STORY OF BENJAMIN:
"LIFE IS TOO SHORT TO BE IN A HURRY"

Benjamin was a successful engineer and inventor who suffered a catastrophic accident at work.

The real pain started when the accident happened. I was at work. I'm going downstairs and the janitor had mopped the floors—very slippery when they're wet tile floors. I hit that thing and injured my neck, my right shoulder, my left shoulder, my wrists, my low back—all up and down my back, tore tendons in my left ankle, suffered knee damage, and so on. I ended up with a reactive arthritis to a point where I was absolutely crippled. I couldn't move, my body hurt so badly. The pain was terrible—I've never experienced anything like that, and it wouldn't go away. I was living on morphine, and the pain never went away. All the drugs did was make it so I didn't care about it. It detached my mind from the pain. The pain was still there, but I didn't care about it anymore.

Here was the big turning point for me with the pain. One day, while I was in bed, I was listening to some music. I felt as if I was becoming detached from my body—that is, the me, the essence of my thinking, my soul, my consciousness became detached—and I was sort of floating around throughout the universe. I was every-where at once and nowhere in particular—that's the only way I can describe it. It was a very curious feeling, a very comfortable feeling, like your whole essence is being scattered everywhere, just like the hydrogen gas in the universe. I eventually came to realize—as I sort of reintegrated, you might say—that I need to go into music; that is the healthiest thing for me, the most nurturing thing for me. I'd had enough of engineering.

Since I had that spiritual revelation or whatever, it let me accept the pain. It was almost a Zenlike acceptance of the pain. The pain is not something I can ignore, it's not something I can fight, it's not something I would ever expect to be free of. It's going to be my con-stant companion through life, whether I like it or not. It's going to be there, so I need to come to terms with it and accept that it's going to be there, have it very clear in my mind what its role is and what its dangers are and what my role is and what my strengths are and where my weaknesses are. So it became that kind of an acceptance. If there wasn't that intense pain, I never would've had that experi-ence. I'm convinced of that.

Later in the interview, Benjamin remembers what he had been think-ing about just before he had his experience listening to music.

I was lying in bed before I had this revelation or whatever you want to call it. And I said to myself, *You know life is not worth living if it's going to be like this. The doctors say that I'm never going to get any better. It's just going to get worse and worse. And I can't take this any-more, I just can't do this.* And I felt totally helpless, and then I started thinking: *How can I solve this problem?* One way was to end it. So I planned my exit strategy. Just take an overdose of the morphine. Clean, simple—I had it there. I had enough to kill a horse. And once I said, *Okay, that's a good exit strategy and I'm at peace with it,* then I felt as if a burden had been lifted, as if I now had some measure of control over my life. Even if it was to end it, I had a way of conquering the pain. It never came close to that, but soberly, honestly thinking about it, and accepting the fact that this is something I could do, gave me a sense of freedom—an enlightened feeling, so to speak. I can't find the words to describe the feelings. *I finally thought, I'm going to really do something with music.*

I was able to start moving about. I would go and volunteer to be an usher for concerts. Here I am with crutches, leg braces, wrist braces, and I'm greeting people and I'm doing the tickets. I just felt so good to be in that environment. I do a whole lot of stuff in exchange for the lessons that I take. I still have those medications available, but I rarely take them. The thing is, most of the time I don't think about it. Like when I'm playing the piano. What worked for me was to have a real passion about music. I'm just still in awe of the thing. I had learned meditation years before that, and I think that helped me. But I hadn't practiced it regularly for maybe twenty years—you get busy with your career. Life's too short to be in a hurry. I've learned that.

When Benjamin planned to take an overdose of morphine if his pain became intolerable, he regained a sense of control. This decision can also be viewed as a way of accepting his mortality. The existential reality of death is often avoided or denied and is thought to be the basic source of human anxiety (Becker 1997). Many physicians and those with chronic pain stories describe facing their human vulnerability and limitations and gaining strength through accepting the fragility of life. After Benjamin planned his "exit strategy," a burden was lifted; he had a sense of freedom and enlightenment. His revelation while listening to music was an experience of universal unity or oneness, followed by a clear and decisive acceptance of his pain and the decision to develop his lifelong passion for music.

We observed the themes of letting go and acceptance intertwined in many of the participants who chose the path to wisdom. The basic desire for healing and meaning is a powerful force that keeps people moving on the path, even though it may take many years to accept a trauma. Putting the experience out of awareness is balanced by the motivation to bring the experience into consciousness, accept it, and ultimately integrate it into a more meaningful life.

The psychologist Richard Lazarus wrote about the process of coping well with distress, and his words very aptly describe what we saw in many of our participants. He observed that people who cope effectively tend to "expand the envelope" (2006, 20) by venturing beyond where they have gone before to reach the limits of what is possible. Although this action adds to their stress, the challenge of doing so makes life more gratifying. Dr. H gained much satisfaction by being an attentive listener to other physicians struggling to accept their mistakes. Benjamin left engineering to develop his lifelong passion for music. As Lazarus explains:

> Stress is, in effect, not necessarily a negative force. It can mobilize us to achieve more than we believed could be accomplished, and it can even lead to a greater appreciation of life. From crisis, too, can come a reorganization of our lives in ways that leave us more productive, engaged, and satisfied than before the crisis. (2006, 20)

Expanding the envelope involves accepting the unfamiliar into your life, which some people find difficult. When the unfamiliar is also very painful, the stress can be overwhelming and lead most of us, at least initially, to turn away. Lazarus draws attention to the balance between the stress and the gratification that can come from accepting painful experiences.

We studied the personality traits associated with those who showed a strong ability to accept their pain and talk about their experiences in positive ways. These personality traits shed light on why, for some people, it may be easier to accept and cope with adverse circumstances. As you might expect, the personality data indicate that people who are predisposed to good moods rather than bad moods have an advantage in accepting. But other traits are also associated with working through adversity.

OPENNESS TO EXPERIENCE

People who chose the path of wisdom scored high in "openness to experience," a trait of people who enjoy expanding the envelope. Previous studies show that openness to experience is associated with wisdom. In our study, most of the participants scored high in openness, especially the pain patients who exemplified the qualities of wisdom. Their lives reflected the many facets of openness, including the capacity to accept and approach their pain by exploring different ways of healing. A strong creative spirit resonated through their narratives and expressed itself in the visual arts, music, and a love of nature, as well as a strong desire to better themselves and help others. Some were long-term practitioners of yoga and meditation and said that this background and training helped in accepting, healing, and living well with pain. These participants can serve as positive role models for those who are less adventurous by nature. Seeing the success of others paves the way and makes it easier for those who are not as open to trying something new. We can learn to be more open and optimistic through experience.

Lenn, who had been meditating for almost thirty years, worked through her debilitating pain following a car accident. She energetically describes her ability to accept and alleviate her pain "using her different techniques," and also tells what she experiences when she says, "No!"

> There have been certain times in my life when I've experienced pain, and you want to go "No, no, no" to the pain. That just increases the pain. But the more you can accept it, first mentally, and then start using different techniques, the more you find the pain subsiding.
>
> So you have to surrender to it if you want to get through it. That's what I've found. You have to surrender to the experience. The more you fight it, the worse it becomes, because not only are you having

a physical experience, now you're having a mental and emotional experience, which seems to increase the negative physical experience. So if you're able to surrender, it's as if you're telling yourself, *Yes. I am most definitely in pain right now, but mentally and emotionally, I'm fine.* And so it decreases the level at which you're experiencing discomfort. It's as if you're accepting, *Yeah, I'm in physical discomfort right now, but I know that at some point it will pass.*

Others echoed these ideas. Tracey DeGregory, who appears in *Choosing Wisdom*, started to get migraines as a child. Her condition worsened until her headaches were nearly relentless as a young adult. She contrasts the effects of resistance and acceptance.

I resisted life and made my pain worse because I feared the pain or refused to accept it. I learned that acceptance and resignation are two different things, and sometimes, in the short term, surrendering to pain is the best thing you can do.

Mary became ill with malaria while visiting the tropics forty years ago. Her lengthy recovery was followed by a painful condition that eventually was diagnosed as fibromyalgia.

I've always been an open-minded person, so that may be part of it, but if you allow yourself to let that sink in and accept it, it's easier to deal with, and I think that's where wisdom comes from.

Sam is a mosaic artist who developed carpal tunnel syndrome from the repetitive strain of cutting and working with tile. The severe pain in his wrists interrupted his work in the middle of a fulfilling career. Sam grapples with the paradox of acceptance and letting go.

Part of it for me was letting go because I was holding it in. Holding it in is, in reality, not accepting your condition, and I've accepted my condition. Letting go was taking control and saying, *I have to help myself.* You ultimately have to take control.

The power that pain has is to tell your body to heal itself, but then you have to release it. If you hold it in, it's going to hurt more— acceptance and then the release, acceptance and then release. I think that if you channel that energy through your breath, that will help you to get a rhythm going so that it's like your heartbeat, and it's like your blood that flows through. It comes and it goes.

This subtle distinction may not make immediate sense to you. Accept it *and* release it? The breath work Sam describes offers a practical way to understand this. Breathing in and accepting good, clean air and then releasing carbon dioxide is a process we do continuously in order to live. Accept the positive, release the negative. Mindful breathing techniques are an age-old, universal way to relieve stress and harmonize the body, mind, and spirit. We heard many stories of breathing through the pain.

Lenn, Tracey, Mary, and Sam all scored very high in openness and all seemed to be naturals at the practice of mindful breathing to accept and release pain. Taking a closer look at practices that use the mind to relieve stress sheds further light on acceptance. Mindfulness can be a powerful ally in living through and releasing intensely painful experiences. The quiet observer in each of us can be aware that we are suffering terribly while the observer itself is not suffering and offers a place of peace and acceptance. Cultivating the ability to shift to a place of pure awareness provides both immediate relief from suffering and a way to integrate and heal our painful experiences.

Acceptance can be cultivated in the practice of meditation and mindfulness. Chapter 11 explores these techniques in more detail. Mindfulness is described as an awareness of present experience with acceptance, and the state of being fully present without habitual reactions (Greeson, Brantley, and Didonna 2009). Our habitual reactions, in the face of adversity, are often the distress and painful feelings noted earlier. The nature of mindfulness is one of a gentle and loving acceptance that has the power to transform an unwanted experience into something of value and interest.

ACCEPTING RESPONSIBILITY

The physicians in our study describe the process of acceptance as a calm acknowledgment of responsibility, releasing thoughts or feelings about being a "bad" doctor. Acceptance is a quiet and powerful state in which negative thoughts and feelings are released and attention is turned to the positive.

Dr. M struggled for years after his patient died from complications following a liver transplant. He came to accept and "quietly own" that he made a wrong decision about a patient.

> Probably the slowest part of it was the quiet recognition that the buck does stop here. You are going to make wrong decisions frequently and the job is to make sure you truly just own that as a part of the passion for your job. I am not bad—this is part of it. Nobody ever talked about this kind of stuff when we were going through medical school.

Dr. J is a general surgeon whose patient developed complications during surgery and died during her attempt to resuscitate him. Poor communication among the team was partly responsible for this unexpected and tragic outcome.

> Acceptance is big. I spent most of my life saying, "I'll be happy when I achieve this," "I'll be happy when I get that," "I'll be happy when. . ." It took me a long time to figure out that I have everything right now, everything I need. Learning that lesson was hard, so acceptance is very important. I focus on doing the best job I can possibly do, but then the outcome is out of my control. I learned to accept what my outcome is, and I don't deal with the anxiety and all the negative feelings that go with that.

Openness, Release, Empowerment, and Choosing a Better Life

Although the stories we have heard differ in their details, there are some clear commonalities. As Dr. H says, the reaction to having the rug pulled out from under you is universal, and what he experienced does not just apply to medical situations. Both Benjamin and Dr. H use the same words—"a burden being lifted"—to describe the release of bottled-up distress. This release is empowering, often giving a feeling of responsibility and control in the midst of facing our limitations and human mortality. Benjamin and Dr. H each scored high on openness, and this trait may have contributed to Benjamin's unusual experience with music and Dr. H's willingness to talk with others about his experience. Talking helped Dr. H turn toward his experience and face the reality that life sometimes goes terribly wrong and bad things happen. He stopped having flashbacks and started to approach his experience actively by taking care of others in similar circumstances.

The importance of positive influences cannot be overstated, whether it is a support group, relaxation techniques, mindfulness, or music. Benjamin and Dr. H valued a virtuous life: Benjamin had become fed up with the lack of ethics in his engineering job, and Dr. H developed a deep desire to help others in need. The drive to be a better person, to give to others, and to discover meaning in life is a powerful motivation that we observe in those who choose to let go of negative feelings, accept their circumstances, and move through adversity.

A Step Taken Many Times

Acceptance is a major step along the path of wisdom, as illustrated in the experiences described in this chapter. But a chapter on acceptance would not be complete without recognizing that feelings of deep acceptance can sometimes fade when the struggle to fully deal with the reality sets in. To paraphrase Sam, as we progress along the path, there is a rhythm like a heartbeat: it comes and it goes, accepting and releasing.

We can sometimes accept the unacceptable and love the unlovable, but then fall back into enduring distress.

Pain patients often talk about good days and bad days. On some days their pain is at a minimum or they are even pain-free, and on other days the pain is intense and unrelenting. Most people can relate. Natural fluctuations in emotional and physical distress are often concentrated in a really bad day, or a difficult time can persist for weeks. Pain patients often remind themselves that even though they may feel miserable at the moment, the pain will not last. They've learned not to give in to a woe-is-me state of mind and to take steps to improve their mood and outlook. They often had lists of things to do, ready at hand, to help themselves feel better: take a walk in the woods, talk to a friend, listen to music, meditate, take a bath, do something nice for someone else, light a candle, put their feet up, or conjure up a positive memory. Anything that helps ease distress also helps bring back feelings of well-being and acceptance. Pam, who is featured in the documentary, lived through a lengthy recovery after a bad fall on the ice. In the extra features we see her office lined with Post-it Notes of inspiration to help her get through discouraging days: "This too shall pass." Like many of the other pain patients, Pam takes a forewarned-is-forearmed attitude toward bad days. Remembering that the bad days will pass gets easier with practice, and having a list of ways to feel better helps.

This struggle may be harder for some people than others due to a disposition for negative moods or a childhood history that fostered anxiety, depression, or anger. Some of the pain patients suffered severe childhood trauma and struggled with forgiveness.

Leih was born with a congenital defect in her legs that led to a long series of hospitalizations and surgeries that separated her from her parents. We now understand the trauma of this for a child, and efforts are made to keep close connections with parents whenever possible. Leih has cultivated a deep acceptance of her pain and of herself, and she describes the cycle of learning with forgiving and accepting herself.

I've become more of a forgiving person over time, and that has been one of those growth areas that I've consciously worked on. I think one of the things I've learned is you really have to be able to forgive yourself. In living, no one is perfect and you make mistakes. I find that with those kinds of things, like forgiveness, you never learn a lesson completely all the way through once. You continue to learn it with more depth over time as you continue to experience whatever it is. So I've had kind of an ongoing bout with learning how to forgive myself and others.

Like many other participants, Leih looks at temporary setbacks as an opportunity for learning. In the same fashion, we can look at the struggle with dark moods and acceptance as offering a potential for growth rather than an impediment. In the documentary's extra features, Tracey describes the process of reframing—turning a negative into a positive through a change in perspective. Realizing that we can improve our emotional well-being through a conscious shift in perspective and by taking steps toward a positive outlook can be an empowering experience. The wide-angle point of view reframes adversity, from suffering to taking steps on the path to wisdom.

Is it possible to sustain acceptance in the stress and strain of daily life? Wisdom scholars describe the cultivation of detachment. "Wise people struggle to let go of worldly passions and anxieties while remaining engaged in the world" (Achenbaum 2004, 301). The aspirations of wise people sound very much like the definitions of mindfulness, a lifelong practice and discipline. Like the other steps along the path, acceptance is a step taken not once but many times. It is indeed a struggle, with times of acceptance giving us the respite and inspiration to continue on the way.

5. Stepping In

Optimism is a strategy for making a better future. Because unless you believe that the future can be better, you are unlikely to step up and take responsibility for making it so. —NOAM CHOMSKY

CONFUCIUS SAID that a journey of a thousand miles begins with a single step, and there couldn't be a more appropriate overview of this chapter. The first response of people facing adversity is often to back away or try to avoid what has happened. Many struggle with feeling helpless, overwhelmed by their circumstances, and powerless to change them. Others disengage from trying to cope altogether and practice forms of denial or distraction; they just give up. At some point, however, those people who were able to move forward in a positive way were able to move beyond helplessness to empowerment. Participants described an active move in taking charge, or *stepping in* to their experience.

This notion of "stepping in" is in many ways a familiar part of our culture. How many times have we encouraged our children, ourselves, or our friends or colleagues to do this? "Step up and face the music." "Take your medicine." "Take charge." "Take it like a man." "Shoulder on." Or even the latest version, "Put on your big-girl pants." This notion of stepping in, however, goes beyond accepting the consequences of our actions or the kind of acceptance examined in the previous chapter. What we've termed "stepping in" refers to an often conscious decision to take action—actions that in our study included taking responsibility, disclosure, apology, learning what happened, and doing the right thing. This phenomenon of actively engaging with the trauma, or stressor, has been demonstrated in numerous other research reports. For example, studies of how U.S. citizens coped in the aftermath of the attacks on September 11, 2001, found that those who just gave up trying to work through the trauma of the events fared worse overall than those who engaged in active coping strategies. Roxane Cohen Silver and her colleagues were interested in determining what factors affected the ability of a nationwide sample of Americans to adjust after the terrorist attacks. They found that "actively coping in the immediate aftermath of the attacks was the only strategy that appeared to be protective against ongoing distress" (Silver et al. 2002). Another 9/11 study conducted by Crystal Park and her colleagues suggested that "actively engaging with a stressor" and even being "aroused by anger" make posttraumatic growth more likely (Park et al. 2008).

An Australian study of patients who had suffered traumatic injury from accidents also tried to determine what factors or behaviors facilitated growth. Most of these study participants felt that their accident experience was a "springboard for growth that enabled them to develop new perspectives on life and living" (Turner and Cox 2004, abstract). What helped them reach this point in their recovery? The study authors, de Sales Turner and Helen Cox, identified a theme they called "staying resolute." They explain that "each [patient] had, within the first year of their rehabilitation process, decided that they would face their journey towards recovery positively. They determined they would somehow find the strength to keep a positive attitude in order to face what lay ahead and keep working to their goal" (6).

This related to the phenomenon of willpower, with the participants using words such as "determination," "motivation," and "stubbornness" to describe their willpower. Each one had, within the first year of the rehabilitation process, decided that they would face their journey toward recovery positively. They determined that they would somehow find the strength to keep a positive attitude in order to face what lay ahead and keep working toward their goal.

One patient said she was depressed initially, "but then she 'took charge' and became determined" (9). In a study of men who had been given a prostate cancer diagnosis, researchers found that emotional distress was more likely among those who used avoidant coping, denial, or behavioral disengagement (Perczek et al. 2002).

It's hard to imagine the anguish that Dr. C felt when she learned that she had failed to diagnose her patient's lung cancer. She thought she might have to quit practicing medicine. *I can't be a doctor anymore*, she thought. *I don't want to hurt people. I want to help people.* Although the patient's oncologist assured Dr. C that the two- or three-month delay in the diagnosis wasn't going to have an impact on how well the patient did, Dr. C didn't feel any better. *How many other mistakes have I made that I don't know about?* she wondered. She was too ashamed to tell her colleagues, afraid that they would think she wasn't up to standards and that she wasn't a good enough doctor to care for their patients.

When she broke the terrible news to her patient, he was justifiably angry and upset. "How could you do this to me? I'm going to die now because you didn't follow up on this fast enough."

For over a month, Dr. C followed her patient's progress from a distance. She stayed in touch with the oncologist as the patient underwent cancer treatments. Finally she realized that she needed to apologize to him. "It took all the courage I could muster to go back and see him," she said. "I thought he was just going to lash out at me again, but I felt such a strong need to ask him to forgive me and to check on him and to let him know that I care about him and that I would never mean him any harm." Standing outside his hospital door that day, seeking his forgiveness, she was certain that this was the hardest thing she'd ever done.

She went into his room, filled that morning with his family members, and before she could even say a word, he told her he was so happy to see her and so touched that she had come to visit. "I know that you care about me," he said, and he even apologized for being so angry with her before. His family told her that he spoke so often about how she took such good care of him.

Seeking forgiveness from her patient allowed Dr. C to take that first step toward healing. It was a long and difficult journey for her, but ultimately she became more sensitive and alert to the privilege of her profession. "From then on it made me much more awed at the power that physicians do have, and to be very respectful of that. And not to take it for granted."

What Does Stepping in Look Like?

We called this element of moving through adversity "stepping in" because that's exactly what it resembles. It's a movement forward, often slow and halting, other times bold and assertive. It's a movement through the trauma and toward healing. For pain patients, this step forward often signified a shift from frustration or passive resignation to taking charge of their own circumstances. Sometimes it was as simple as changing or reframing a question. For example, a patient might ask, *What can I do to help myself?* rather than, *Why can't my doctor make the pain go away?* Or *How am I responsible?* instead of *Who's to blame?* Other times more concrete decisions and actions are involved, such as seeking out a new therapy or treatment. For physicians who had made a mistake, stepping in often involved facing the patient or family, explaining honestly what had happened, and apologizing for the result. Many times, patients and physicians could move forward by gleaning new knowledge; patients might take more responsibility for their treatments, and doctors might investigate what went wrong so that it would never happen again. In both cases, becoming an expert either in self-care or in a particular medical condition or procedure was the key to moving ahead. The common thread, however, was a shift or movement from a passive stance to an active, exploratory stance.

Stepping in also mirrors the metaphor of putting one foot in front of the other as a way to move through difficult times. For some individuals, stepping in simply entailed getting out of bed each day and moving forward, one step at a time. When things are terrible, that's about as much as you can expect. One patient, Mary Anne, who suffered terrible pain from a surgical error, described forcing herself "to push through it" in order to live her life more fully. "I was very active growing up. I love being a mom, love being a wife, love owning my own business, love being a grandma. I felt like I wasn't participating in my own life.

I just had to push through it. I don't care if I hurt." Although her pain continued, by gradually reengaging in her life and the roles she cherished, she eventually began to feel more gratitude and less anger toward her circumstances. Another patient, Maurice, who tells his story in the film, advises others with pain to take baby steps:

> First they have to accept the fact that they're going to have pain, but they also have to start believing that they can start taking action to control the pain. And that doesn't always necessarily mean running to the medicine cabinet and popping some pills. It can be something, I don't want to say small, because exercise for people can be a huge, major factor, a big challenge for them. So, it could be something . . . they need to start believing that they can start taking control of the pain and taking some baby steps. You know what I'm saying—taking some baby steps to deal with that pain. But just accept it. It's here to stay, and you have two choices. Either conquer it or let it kick your behind for the rest of your life.

For some, the stepping in may have been the result of fate or even someone else's doing, perhaps someone encouraging an action that would ultimately begin the healing process. Another way to understand this process is to consider those who struggle with addiction. Not only does the one-day-at-a-time mantra resonate with the need to move in a forward direction, the notion of taking that first important step—to treatment and toward recovery—is a powerful example of the importance of stepping in.

Dr. J, the surgeon whose patient died a preventable death on the operating table, became addicted to the painkiller Percocet. "I just didn't want to feel anything anymore," she said. Later she added Valium to the mix. She needed the drugs just to "be normal." But then it all came crashing down, putting her job and even her family in jeopardy.

> And there was that moment. It's when you realize what you have done. That is when you have what for me was a moment of clarity.

And for me it all came together in the middle of the night. I said, "I first have to address this addiction before I do anything, and then I've got to address this grief. I can't keep living this way. This has to change." And then it was the very next morning I got on the phone and started making arrangements.

Captain of the Ship: Taking Responsibility

For some in our study, stepping in involved taking responsibility for their circumstances. For patients, that often meant reducing their reliance on medicine and physicians and increasing their reliance on their own power to make changes. For physicians, it often meant taking responsibility for what went wrong, for their patients and for their medical team. In the film *Choosing Wisdom* Dr. Andy Wolf shares the tragic story of a patient who died in the hospital. It was a sudden and unexpected death that left everyone on his care team stunned and devastated. "It was a tragedy for everybody, having this horrible, horrible thing happen." But in the immediate aftermath, he felt an overwhelming sense that he was the "captain of the ship," and that he needed to maintain order and stability for everyone involved.

> I very quickly got the team together in a room and said, "We have to accept that we have had a tragedy here. We're not sure what happened, but let's process it." I just had everybody process it right there.

The focus of that gathering and much of the time in the following days was to process the event emotionally. The medical processing would come later, but for now, Dr. Wolf felt it was important to "try to turn this into a growth experience from the start." After the initial tears and sadness, the result was a team that responded in a healthy way, without defensiveness, blaming, casting aspersions, or anger. Upon reflection, Dr. Wolf believes that the moment of bringing everyone together "was probably the turning point, right there. The rest of it sort of fell into place after that." In the immediate aftermath, they were able to pull together to care for the family and themselves, and to focus on how to prevent a similar occurrence in the future. "I feel like the resident physicians came through it, as far as I can tell, without denial of what had happened, but also not feeling like terrible people—that they are incompetent, terrible people." Dr. Wolf says that his leadership had come from a combination of his personal and professional maturity, and learning "how to handle tragic events in one's life that I had evolved to the point where I could handle it in real time pretty, pretty well."

Fake It until You Make It

For patients, stepping in often involves a move away from helplessness toward taking responsibility and reclaiming control. Lauren suffered from debilitating migraines for over fifteen years before she began to see any improvement. For her, showing compassion for herself was the first step toward healing, but it didn't come naturally.

> I think the physical pain made me really judgmental of myself—that I was weak, why is this happening to me: I'm not perfect. So I go on this attack of myself, which just brings more anxiety and just kind of like a vicious circle. And I just had to stop. It doesn't feel natural for me to be compassionate with myself, but it's kind of like you fake it until you make it so it's become like a practice. I don't necessarily believe it, but I've got to do something because it's depressing or I feel powerless if I don't take control.

For patients in our study who had tried traditional therapies with minimal results, stepping in began when they made a conscious decision to explore their options, often trying something new, such as meditation, yoga, or energy healing. Patricia suffered from fibromyalgia so severe that at one point she was on six different medications, none of which relieved her symptoms. She tried spinal injections. Nothing worked. She couldn't sleep, hold a book, or sit at her computer. Finally, she had had enough.

> Rather than going to go see doctors, I thought, *This is nonsense—I can't be a patient my whole life. I am going to be somebody who takes control of it—be a person who has fibromyalgia rather than be fibromyalgia*—and that's why I thought that I've got to get off the medications. Going to doctors, physical therapy, it seemed to help short term, but long term did nothing. That is why I started going to yoga.

DISCLOSURE AND APOLOGY

For the physicians, the element of stepping in sometimes meant not only actively taking responsibility for the error that had occurred but also having the courage to face devastated patients and families. This often resulted in the process of disclosure, or talking honestly with the patient or family about what happened. As seen in Dr. C's story when she told her patient about his delayed diagnosis, this encounter can be extremely difficult. Disclosure is a very complex process involving multiple layers and many reasons why it takes courage.

The first layer is the legal system. Although not as common a practice as it was a decade ago, lawyers have traditionally instructed doctors to keep silent, with the concern that disclosing or apologizing to a patient will result in a lawsuit. Therefore, many doctors struggle with errors that could easily have remained hidden from the patient. What if an error was made that had no adverse outcome? Should the doctor disclose to the patient in that situation? A doctor may think, *If I tell you about what I did, you may sue me for something you wouldn't have known about if I hadn't told you.* Yet many doctors adhere to a code that requires them to do the right thing even at risk to themselves.

Dr. Q delayed his diagnosis of a patient's pancreatic cancer; the patient, an eighty-eight-year-old woman, died. Although an earlier diagnosis would not have changed the ultimate outcome, he felt compelled to speak to the family, to tell the woman's family about the delay in identifying her disease as cancer. Said Dr. Q,

> Keeping stuff inside festers and feels really bad and really dishonest. Confession is important to me. It would have been okay if they had been furious with me. It would have been well within their rights also.

Many doctors agree with this approach of facing the family rather than hiding and holding onto secrets. One insisted on talking with his patient's family, against the legal advice from the hospital.

> I felt like the right thing to do was to go talk to them and tell them what had happened. And if they felt like they needed to sue me, then we would just have to deal with that.

Another layer of, or barrier to, disclosure is the shame in having made a mistake. We all have felt the shame of making an error, but few of us have made a mistake that resulted in someone's death or injury. Physicians who have erred must face their patients, their colleagues, themselves, and sometimes lawyers and lawsuits, and many physicians in this position carry the weight of this shame for years. Dr. C's shame kept her locked in silence at a time when she most needed the support of her peers.

> I was too ashamed to tell any of my colleagues, so I suffered in silence for probably a week or two. Because, I thought, *if I tell them, they're not going to trust me to cover their patients, they're not going to think I'm smart anymore*—all of those things go through your head. I mean, you really feel defective, you feel like you're not up to standards.

A third layer of disclosure is the doctor's realization that revealing the error could result in a broken relationship with one's patient. In the best doctor-patient relationships, an intimacy and caring develop, often over the course of many years and the highs and lows of a patient's health history. Just as a patient would be saddened by the loss of this relationship, so, too, would a doctor. Dr. T is an ob-gyn who enjoys her close relationships with her patients, their newborn babies, and their families. She often cares for patients through multiple pregnancies and "really significant events in their life." Living in a small town, she enjoys watching the babies she's delivered grow up. For her, one of the hardest aspects of an error during childbirth and the ensuing lawsuit was the destruction of her relationship with her patient.

> We had a really good relationship before this. I delivered her first child, too, and watched her deal with some pretty difficult stuff during this second pregnancy. I think probably her mother and certain family members pushed her into the lawsuit. There's very little available for a special-needs child, so this is the American mechanism to make this happen. But based on her deposition, I don't think she was really angry with me.

Dr. T remembers that she and the patient even shared a smile over an inside joke during the hearing.

Another physician, Dr. D, had a similar experience with a delayed diagnosis. Shortly after the correct diagnosis was revealed, she was invited to attend an event that the patient and his family also attended. Several physicians were in the patient's family, and one of them asked, "How could you miss that?" Dr. D told another family member, a family physician like herself, that she wished more than anything she'd done the ultrasound when the patient had complained of stomach pain the year before. He told her, "Our lives are full of shoulda coulda woulda." His attempt at kindness was helpful, but "it was definitely a hard place to go. I felt like whatever I got, I would deserve. But I stood there. I stood there."

Standing there and listening to the anger of a distraught patient or family member, or waiting outside a patient's hospital door with the intent of seeking forgiveness, is rarely, if ever, easy. Both acts require exceptional courage and resolve. Dr. Jo Shapiro, speaking in the film, talks about facing her patient following a surgical error. She explained everything to him and his family. She apologized. She was very careful to tell him exactly what happened and what their plans were to repair the damage. It was helpful to be able to face him and explain it all to him. "That said," she reflects, "all of those feelings of being very, very sad about what happened would bubble up and would make it hard for me to even want to go in the room and see him." Overcome with feelings of inadequacy, she remembers forcing herself to visit him twice a day. "Every part of me was saying, *Don't go in there. It will just remind me of all that went wrong.*" But ultimately she realized, "I didn't want my emotions and my needs to get in the way of helping him get through this process."

Approaching the patient and the family rather than avoiding them is a critical step in healing. An experienced physician, Dr. G, accidentally gave her patient too much medication in preparation for a test while in the hospital. The elderly and already fragile patient became unresponsive and had to be resuscitated. Dr. G, who immediately went to the patient's waiting children to report what she had done, underscored the importance of facing the family in this healing process. She points out,

> I would encourage people not to run from this process. I think people don't want to talk about it, but I've never had a bad experience when we've been able to get families back in and talk about unexpected bad outcomes with them. Some physicians want to hide from those meetings, and I try to encourage them not to because it's a way for the families to heal, it's a way for us to heal.

Dr. T, the surgeon, agreed:

> You've got to live with your complications. One of my old attendings taught me that many years ago. When you have a complication, the natural tendency is avoidance. You want to stay away from it with some surrealistic hope that it'll just go away if you ignore it.

But after years of experience, she has concluded,

> As hard as it is, you have to suck it up and you have to walk in
> that room every day and see your patient and take care of her and
> address her needs and get through this just like she's got to get
> through it. And you'll both get better.

Finally, other forms of disclosure do not involve these open conversations with patients. Sometimes doctors are unable to talk with patients
or families, perhaps because the patient has died and has no surviving
family. In these cases, physicians tell us that disclosing to a mentor,
peer, or friend is a helpful form of disclosure. In the film, Dr. Matt
Goodman told us about his stepping in, which enabled him to move
beyond the error to constructive healing. For him, stepping in entailed
telling a trusted colleague about his mistake:

> I think the disclosure was the thing that helped me most. Telling the
> story and just mulling it over. However I processed it, it's just incred-
> ibly painful. Then a couple of days later it's not quite as painful, and
> then I can start to intellectualize and learn about it and figure out
> what concrete steps to take to try to keep it from happening again.

What Went Wrong?

What did I do wrong? As Dr. Goodman explains above, finding an answer
to this question in the aftermath of an error is critical for physicians
as they begin to move toward healing. Many go to a trusted mentor or
an expert who can give them objective feedback. Almost immediately
after the death of a beloved patient, Dr. Q sought out his mentor, whose
counsel was important in helping him process the event. "There was
no confessional or wallowing," he said of his conversation with his
mentor. "But he told me the two essential things. 'Yes, you did wrong,
and yes, this is something to learn from' and 'No, you didn't kill this
person you loved.'" Dr. Q also went immediately to a surgeon for more

information about the patient's case, inviting him to coffee. He said his conversation with the surgeon "wasn't reassuring or nonreassuring." He was an excellent surgeon, he said, not the touchy-feely type, and what he said amounted to, "Yeah, you screwed up, and yeah, you wouldn't have saved her life if you'd ordered a CAT scan the first day." So, in a sense, the conversation was reassuring. "But I didn't want to be reassured. I just needed to talk to somebody about having screwed up."

Sometimes you need to move beyond uncertainty and ambiguity before healing and growth can occur. We saw many physicians and patients step in by becoming experts in whatever realm was important for their situation. For the physicians, it was often a matter of learning "Why did this error happen? How can I be sure this will never happen again?" Dr. T, the surgeon, told us, "I decided, okay, this is how I'm going to deal with this. I said, 'I'm just going to face this head-on, read everything I possibly can about uterine rupture, and become the most knowledgeable person in this subject on the face of the planet.'"

Learning the facts and becoming well versed can also prevent errors from occurring again and allows healing to begin. Said one physician, "If I know that this won't ever happen to another patient, I can begin to forgive myself." One physician offered advice to other doctors who may experience a medical error. He encouraged this knowledge-seeking behavior in order to learn "if you were wrong. If you were wrong, you learn you were wrong, and you change what you're doing. And if you're right, it makes you feel better. It reinforces what you were doing, and you don't change it."

A Problem to Be Solved

Carol spent nearly ten years with such terrible neck pain that she would often lie down wherever she was—on a park bench, on the floor— because she couldn't go on without some relief. Massage made her pain worse. Yoga and meditation didn't work. Acupuncture didn't work either. She spent thousands and thousands of dollars going to doctors and therapists, looking for a source and a cure for her pain.

> My son was about two and a half, three, when this happened, and
> it was very important to me that my life not be revolving around
> the pain. He didn't need a world that was, 'Mom's always in pain.'

She became very frustrated and finally took matters into her own hands.

> What helped me was that I kept saying to myself, *Every problem
> has a solution. You just don't know this one yet.* And that was how I
> reframed everything. I'm intensely curious. Curiosity has been the
> driving force my entire life, so I used that curiosity.

She began researching on the Internet and going to the nearby medical bookstore to sit and read all the books about pain. Eventually she
discovered that she had a rare syndrome that tightens muscles in the
body, a syndrome that she was then able to control with medication.

> To me, researching was fun. I like to do research. I kept my pain over
> here in this corner of my life as a problem to be solved. I'd tell myself,
> *I don't have the answer yet. That doesn't mean it doesn't exist.* It was
> a goal, and it was always like, *Oh, wow! I wonder if this could be the
> answer!* Every time I learned something new.

Sharing the Story

Learning about the error can help other physicians and their patients.
As we see in part 3, sharing the story with others can serve as a powerful teaching and learning tool. Another study physician, Dr. B, who
was a resident at the time of his event, became an expert in a particular
bowel disease following the preventable death of a patient who had the
condition. The disease was relatively rare, and no one had been able
to diagnose it in time for his patient. Shortly after the patient's death,
he began to research the disease. He now considers himself a "minor
expert" on the condition. "That was part of my coping," he said. "To
learn about it and say, 'How can I help other people?'" Twenty years

after the patient's death, Dr. B continues to help other young physicians, having told the story "probably fifty times" and using it as a teaching case so that it doesn't happen to anyone else.

Traditionally, when an error occurs, doctors come together privately to discuss the error in what is known as a morbidity and mortality conference (M&M). The goal of an M&M is to determine what went wrong and how the problem can be fixed. Unfortunately, the tenor of these conferences is not always conducive to discovering why things went wrong and how that particular error could be prevented, and instead can inappropriately focus on finding someone to blame. As a result, we miss opportunities for changing unsafe systems of care, and the stress associated with an M&M creates an atmosphere of shame and guilt when errors occur. Although M&Ms range along a continuum in terms of tone and effectiveness, they are improving. However, even in the best of M&Ms, the emotional impact of the error on the caregivers is rarely discussed. The result is that emotional isolation for the physicians is often the rule rather than the exception.

Support groups or sharing with a trusted colleague or friend can have a powerful impact on the healing process. We heard this numerous times from physicians, most of whom endured a period of silence induced by shame or legal advice. Several physicians, even those whose error had occurred a decade or more ago, admitted that the research interview was the first time they had revealed their experience to anyone besides their spouse.

For others, sharing their story was often the turning point. Finally overcoming shame in order to talk to a trusted colleague is an important step. One physician, Dr. L, talked about being invited to speak about professionalism with several other presenters. Each panel member shared a personal story of coping with a medical error.

> I think the turning point for me was really when we each shared our story. I think that was the most emotionally fraught occasion. I didn't share just a story, I shared the feelings. All feelings came out—all the regret and the loss.

A relatively new movement in medicine acknowledges that physicians do have human feelings and that processing those feelings is vital to maintaining their own wellness. Several doctors talked about being in these small, nurturing groups that encouraged sharing difficult experiences. Dr. H, the pediatric surgeon introduced in chapter 4, talked about the physician support group through which he began his journey toward healing. Until he participated in the group, he was never able to process what had happened or constructively address his grief. He continued having flashbacks until he had the opportunity to talk about the child's death and his role in it. The group was "a way of being listened to," and afterward Dr. H felt the burden begin to lift.

Chronological Time versus Choosing in the Moment

When someone steps in doesn't seem to be as important as that they do it at all. For the physicians, stepping in could happen immediately, such as when Dr. Wolf, featured in the film, brought his team together immediately after the patient's death to help them grieve and process what had happened. In Dr. C's case, she knocked on her patient's door to seek forgiveness over a month after her delayed diagnosis was discovered. For Dr. H, who finally shared his story in a safe, small group, his stepping in occurred eight years after the patient had died. Pain patients talk about suffering for years before stepping into their own healing.

Chronological or relational time is not the issue. Most important is the conscious, mindful choice in the moment: *I will tell my story. I will take control of my healing. I choose to seek help. I will learn from my mistake.* This becomes a step in the process of putting the world back together again in new ways, a way of integrating the pain or the error into whom we have become, as we will see more in the next chapter. For some, spirituality in the broadest sense helps people do the right thing, especially when it's hard. Doctors faced the families to apologize because that's what a good doctor does. For others—like Carol, who put her curiosity to work to solve the problem of her pain—bringing the best parts of oneself to the situation makes stepping in possible.

In the film, Dr. Alan Alfano points out that it is an opportunity to be deliberate about bringing the best parts of himself to the disclosure process:

> We bring to bear who we are. Who we are can be helpful, or it can be detrimental to a particular situation. I try to pick the best of who I am to bring to a situation like that, knowing full well that that's what the patients expect and that's what I expect from myself. So every time we do that, there's a little bit of a struggle. We grow from struggle, from that situation where we've made a mistake and we need to go now and face the person whose care we've messed up. The most important thing is that that patient and the family know that I really do care. To be able to express that without seeming false, I think—to be able to express that without being self-serving—is really important. So we try to look on the qualities and the character and compassion; sometimes it's easy and sometimes it's not. Compassion and attention and forgiveness and mercy, and all of those things that we consider the best part of us—that's what I draw on when walking into a situation like that. And I have to have faith that those positives and those characteristics, those portions of my character, will be helpful at the very least. They may not resolve the situation, they may not make everyone feel great, but it should be a positive influence in whatever situation I find myself.

6. Integration

integration *n* **1.** the act of combining or adding parts to make a unified whole. —*COLLINS ENGLISH DICTIONARY–COMPLETE AND UNABRIDGED*

ONE OF THE most difficult components of moving positively through adversity is the process of integrating this terrible experience and its implications into our understanding of ourselves and our world. We are faced with situations that seem so overwhelmingly bad, situations that so deeply challenge our previous understanding of ourselves, that knowing how to move forward is difficult.

Integrating an experience of adversity often requires us to rework some of our most deeply held beliefs about ourselves and the world. Beneath the surface, there are sometimes massive shifts required in our concepts of ourselves, of God, of our place in the world, and of how the world works. It is confusing and frightening, because we cannot always see what's ahead. Letting go of our understanding of things leaves us vulnerable, with no clear sense of where things are going. In the process of growth from trauma we often have to reconcile seemingly irreconcilable differences that call into question our faith, our sense of justice, our understanding of right and wrong, and our way of making sense of the world.

Our study participants faced just such seemingly irreconcilable situations. "I am a doctor. I am supposed to be helping people. But I have made a mistake that hurt someone. How can I keep practicing?" The pain patients had to face this reality: "There might not be an easy fix for this pain, and I have the rest of my life to lead. How can I go forward?" Participants described a daunting process of integrating their imperfections, their pain, and their mistakes into their understanding of themselves in order to create a new narrative for their lives, one that incorporated these situations into a more expansive understanding of themselves and the world.

NARRATIVE DISRUPTION

Robert Neimeyer, the author of "Re-Storying the Loss: Fostering Growth in the Posttraumatic Narrative" (2006), believes that trauma disrupts our "story," the narrative of our lives, so that we have to restructure that narrative if we are to go on. He describes the various forms of narrative disruption that can occur after trauma, which is a useful framework when considering how people move from this disruption to reintegration. In resilient people, some trauma can be assimilated into the existing narrative in such a way that it does not radically undermine the central themes of their life story. The more expansive our narrative, the less likely that we will be blown off course by an event, but rather be able to take it in stride, incorporating that experience into our broad understanding of life. But when the traumatic event presents a direct challenge to the central components of our life narrative, this assimilation is not possible, and the person has to find ways to adapt and change the narrative in order to integrate this experience.

According to Neimeyer (2006), narrative disruption from adversity can take various forms. The situation may result in a *disorganized* narrative, precipitated by a struggle with radically contradictory images and emotions, and a "massive invalidation of the thematic structure on which one's worldview is premised" (73). One example might be the violent attack on a youth camp in Norway that occurred in 2011. A lone gunman, dressed as a policeman, opened fire on unarmed youth gathered at a summer camp. Norway is a country that perceives itself as an open, trusting, peaceful society. The individual families involved and the entire country struggled with horrific images of senseless violence in a society with a worldview anchored in the belief that the camp—and Norway itself—is a relatively safe place, that people (especially ones wearing a police uniform) can be trusted, and that there is justice in the world.

Trauma can also result in *dissociated* narratives, which Neimeyer (2006) describes as silent stories that resist acknowledgment in the public sphere. This occurs most often in response to events that are socially unacceptable, so that the person involved is unable to openly acknowledge the event. These dissociated narratives play out in the survivor's life through a "harsh and vigilant form of self-monitoring and a continuous need to try to segregate this event that the survivor cannot reveal" (73). Many of the physicians in our study reported this kind of narrative disruption. As we will see below, the shame and guilt associated with a medical error, coupled with a culture of medicine that does not accept such events, results in physicians carrying this dissociated narrative for years, unrevealed and unresolved. Dr. H, who made an error as a young attending, noted that it was not until many years later, when he participated in a group intended to help physicians learn to cope with mistakes, that he shared that experience, and only then in an anonymous format. But when he did, even those many years later, he found it enormously helpful. "That was really important to me because when I was able to say that everyone felt the same. That's when I really started to feel better about it."

A third form of narrative disruption occurs when the traumatic event creates a *dominant* narrative, in which the event essentially comes to define the person, blocking out entirely the narrative of who that person was before the event. Another way to describe this is what is commonly called the "victim mentality," in which a person's life becomes defined or dominated by the event. Many of the patients in our study reported struggling with this dominant narrative for years, feeling that their lives were completely consumed by their pain, and their self-concept engulfed by being a pain patient.

Tim is a law enforcement officer. He injured his back when he fell down a ravine in pursuit of a criminal. He struggled with severe back pain for years without significant relief from conventional medical interventions, including many different medications. It all just seemed to make him feel worse. Tim concluded that he didn't want his life to be dominated by his struggle with pain, and he began to take steps to move away from this victim mentality. At that point he began to feel better.

Each type of narrative disturbance that Neimeyer describes—the disorganized narrative, the dissociated narrative, and the dominant narrative—presents different challenges to integration of the event into a new, more expansive, more resilient narrative.

How exactly do people integrate these difficult circumstances? What challenges to their worldview do they have to face, and how do they respond? The ways that people integrate these events depends, in part, on the specific circumstance of the event, and in part on the type of narrative disturbance that the event caused. But obvious themes emerged in the kinds of challenges to integrating these events that patients and doctors faced and the ways in which they successfully negotiated those challenges.

Mistakes, Forgiveness, and Dealing with Imperfection

For the physicians, integrating their mistake into their understanding of themselves as doctors means being able to integrate their humanness into their concept of a doctor; this step is key to moving forward. Somehow they have to accept their imperfections and their humanness and allow themselves to be forgiven, but at the same time not lower the standards to which they hold themselves. Actions on the physician's part may include never forgetting the mistake, learning from the mistake, atoning for it, and making changes to prevent future harm. The more expansive personal narratives contained this acceptance of imperfection as well as the continued striving to be the best possible doctor.

For some physicians, accepting their humanness and their imperfections was extremely difficult, in part because of the unimaginable vulnerability that implied. The idea that they, through their humanity, might be exposing patients to harm was unacceptable.

One young physician related that in his residency he was in the midst of trying to resuscitate a patient during a code. The intravenous central line that he inserted went too deep, puncturing the vein through and through. Unbeknownst to him, all the fluids and blood they were giving to resuscitate the patient ended up going into the retroperitoneum rather than the vein. The patient survived, but the doctor was devastated. He had to stop practicing medicine for a while in order to come to grips with the error he had made.

> I actually stepped away from clinical medicine for two years after residency—not necessarily because of this incident, but just because I didn't know how to be an imperfect physician.

Dr. I is known as a knowledgeable, careful, compassionate physician who misdiagnosed a patient who presented with shortness of breath. Dr. I expressed the ever-present worry that at some point, if something terrible happened, she wouldn't be able to be a doctor anymore.

> There's too much uncertainty about what you do, and too many decisions that need to be made every day. Even if you are really good—and let's say you are good 98 percent of the time—that means you are going to make six or eight wrong decisions a day. Some of those are going to trickle down into something bad; I don't think you can get away from that. I think my career is going well, but at the same time, not very far from the surface is a realization that things could go wrong that I don't see coming and that would prompt me to say, "I really shouldn't be doing this job." I could make a little money, or have a lot of debt or whatever, but if I hurt somebody else or feel ashamed of what I've done, that is undermining to the point that I just won't do it in the long run.

Dr. B related a funny story that helps him to get some perspective on his struggle with perfection. As he explains it, a colleague of his was "festering over something that was going on with a patient."

The next patient came in—it was some country guy—and he said, "You look kind of down, Doc," and he said, "Oh, I'm just not sure I'm doing the right thing with this other situation, and I just feel like I may have messed up." And the guy said, "Doc, you're trying to be perfect—that's the devil talking. The only person who is perfect is the Lord, and when I start feeling that way I just say, "Devil get behind me, devil get behind me, three times, and then I just walk away." I like that.

Successful integration often involves self-forgiveness and acceptance of imperfections, but with an important caveat that makes it more difficult. The physicians are keenly aware that they cannot, must not, ever forget what happened nor in any way lower their standards or let themselves off the hook.

Dr. C, whom we introduced in chapter 5, talked about her struggle with the idea of forgiveness. When asked about that, she said,

One of the biggest problems that I've seen in myself and my colleagues is guilt when we make a mistake. How do you get rid of that guilt? To think that you've hurt someone is just the worst possible thing. But it took a good six months to a year for me to forgive myself.

Dr. X, a very seasoned and well-respected clinician and teacher, who herself missed a diagnosis, reflected on this perception that doctors are perfect and how that perception is reshaped through experience into a more real and truthful perception. As she put it:

One of the processes of growing older and more experienced is that reality replaces icons.

Physicians have to explore ways in which they can accept their imperfections but honor the gravity of their experience and ensure that because of it they become even better doctors. Dr. M struggled for years after one of his patients died following a liver transplant. The circumstances were complex, and the decisions at the time were made difficult by the murky symptoms and signs that the doctor could have attributed to many different illnesses. Nevertheless, when the final correct diagnosis is known through hindsight, the physician is left with the reality that his diagnosis was wrong. Dr. M learned from this experience how to integrate those situations in a way that he felt made him a better doctor and better able to learn from his mistakes. He offered this advice:

> You are going to make wrong decisions frequently. The job is to truly own that as a part of the passion for your job. It sounds strange, but you need to be able to say, "This is not unusual, I am not bad—this is part of it."

We asked Dr. M about whether he can forgive himself:

> I'm working on that one. I think part of me wants to keep that lesson at the forefront.

Dr. L put it this way:

> We make mistakes, we learn from our mistakes, and we have to learn something about resiliency, about fallibility, and about the dangers of holding ourselves to impossible standards. I think wanting to be a better doctor and wanting to do better with the next situation, being honest in a healthy way—I think that's part of being mature.

Dr. V is a surgeon and teaches students and residents. His first experience of a serious error occurred when he was still in training. He is now an attending, and he describes not only keeping the stories of things that have gone wrong over the years constantly present in his mind, but learning to use these stories to teach other physicians how to do things better. As he explains,

I think it honors the memory of those patients if you share these things, if you are willing to carry them with you and never forget.

HUMILITY:
SEEING OURSELVES AS PART OF A WHOLE

One of the ways in which the physicians were able to integrate the reality of their humanness into their concept of being a good doctor was to allow the understanding of their vulnerability to error to inform and influence the way they practiced medicine. Many described how, in the process of learning to accept their limitations, they gained a new appreciation for ways of functioning as a physician that could mitigate the potential for harm. Many of the physicians talked about how they listened more carefully to their colleagues and their patients and relied more on their fellow team members to correct them or to help inform their decisions.

Dr. M reflects on how his experience of a misdiagnosis affected the way he sees things in his everyday work. It is as though his eyes are now open to all the small things that previously went unnoticed, but that are now seen as opportunities to make things better. He talks here about the iterative process of integrating his mistake and his imperfection into a new way of being a physician, one that notices small mistakes, values teams and working together to make things safer for his patients.

> I never thought I was perfect, but, boy, this brought it up big-time. I was trying to quietly own that—noticing those other little errors a little bit more, the little errors that you make all the time that don't matter or somebody else catches them. They still happen. You write the prescription wrong, you call it in wrong, you misread a lab result, think it was okay. Then you realize, *I know I looked at that. Why didn't I notice that that was wrong?* That's just part of our business, and your job is to try to minimize those as much as you can and build in backups.

Moving On: An Increased Sense of Strength, Balance, and Wholeness

For the pain patients, integrating their physical pain into a deeper understanding of themselves allows them to move forward, even if their pain is not resolved. Being able to integrate the possibility that the pain may not subside and allow them to live the kind of life that they hoped to live is crucial. For some, this means making adjustments in their expectations. For many, it means integrating both their pain and a new understanding of their own empowerment into their self-concept.

Maurice, who was injured while in the armed forces, has lived with back pain for several years. He learned how to put his pain in the background in order to go on with his life.

> I'm going to have pain for the rest of my life, whether I want to or not. And I can't let that stop me from living, from trying to enjoy life. I can't let that stop me from whatever goals I have or whatever dreams I have, so I have to look at it like, *Okay, pain, you're with me, but that's okay. When it's time to put you in check, I'm going to put you in check.* That's just pretty much how I look at it.

Many pain patients discover capacities within themselves to reduce the impact of the pain on their lives. A concept of wholeness is an important means of harnessing such capacities. Julie suffers from lesions on the spine and continual pain. She describes how discovering her "core" and having a sense of "wholeness" helped her to move forward even though her pain was not resolved:

> You don't have to have every iota of your illness healed before you can be whole. I came up with this thought that, at my core and at your core, all of us—no matter what's going on—are already whole. Nothing that happens in our lives can get past that core. It bounces

off. Yeah, it might stick us in this joint, that joint, and cause pain. But nothing can destroy your center. Nothing.

Tracey DeGregory described learning to integrate different parts of herself into her whole being. This integrated wholeness is extraordinarily helpful to her in coping with her pain, but she also learned the following from her pain experience:

> We are beings who are physical, emotional, mental, and spiritual. These parts need to be in balance, and if they aren't, we get sick. And figuring out how we are out of balance can provide us with clues that will help us heal or cope.

Many of the pain patients described developing an awareness of the mind/body connection through experiencing the relationship between stress and pain. The pain became an ally in helping them learn to calm the stress response and integrate painful parts of their lives. Instead of becoming more stressed and increasing the pain, they gave positive attention to challenging aspects of their lives.

Julie describes a highly stressful and painful time in her life, when she realized that her emotional trauma was causing her to be in intolerable physical pain. She learned to soothe her pain by engaging the mind/body connection and gradually healed and integrated her past trauma.

> Stress is a terrible factor in pain. I've noticed in the past, when I got highly stressed out, the pain would get very accelerated. There have been times in my life—I remember the pain in my back, and my knees, and my whole body, every joint in my body—I just wanted to put a gun to my head because I was so stressed out. The pain was terrible. So I have learned how to control it with my mind. You have to close your eyes and visualize something that's pleasant to you and put your body there.

Sue felt stressful circumstances in her elbow, which prompted her to look at her circumstances differently.

I know one thing that's very concrete for me has been, especially when the pain in my elbow was ramped up on a daily basis, if I got upset or tense about something, there was no way I wasn't going to feel it in my elbow. I would immediately feel it there. A leads to B. And if I can think about A differently, B will improve.

Maurice put it this way:

There's a connection between stress and pain. When you're stressed, oftentimes your body's talking to you and you might not be paying attention to your body. And it's telling you, because of whatever life challenges you're facing—could be work, could be family, could be personal, could be relational, could be spiritual, whatever the case might be—you're just not in tune with or listening to your body. You're not alert to the messages, the signals your body's giving you.

Achieving this integration of mind, body, and spirit—this whole-ness—isn't an easy process when the physical body is a source of con-stant pain. Tracey described the shift from feeling that her body was an enemy to be fought to being able to partner with her body as an ally.

Making a change in how I viewed my body was really important. My pain initially made me have a negative view of my body. I dis-trusted it, felt as if it had betrayed me, and looked at it mainly as a source of pain, a thing that was keeping me from having a good life. I looked at it more or less as a machine that wasn't working right. I have to say that our culture and the medical profession did much to support that image. (What's the symptom? Here's a pill to pop or a procedure to do to "fix" that symptom.)

As I began exploring alternative practices, I gradually was able to shift to a holistic way of perceiving my body, seeing that it was just as much me as my mind was, that it was my ally instead of my enemy, that it had its own wisdom, that often I just needed to get out of its way so it could heal itself. I came to see that illness is often not about foreign things attacking us from the outside or parts breaking down; rather it's a last-ditch effort to force us to rest if we've been running ourselves into the ground or a way of getting our attention. Once I began cooperating with my body, paying very close attention to subtle cues, having a positive attitude about it, and looking for hidden beliefs and ways I was undermining it, I think I really began to turn a corner and start getting healthier.

Some of the physicians also found that moving through the experience of a medical error gave them an increased sense of their own strength and an increased ability to stand up for the important things in life. It made them more willing to speak up when they felt things were going wrong. These changes also mitigated against future harm.

Dr. B reflected on a situation in which he had a gut feeling that a patient needed urgent surgical attention, but the surgeon disagreed and the surgery was delayed. The patient ultimately died. The decisions involved were all difficult and even hindsight is not always 20/20, but Dr. B felt that he had not advocated forcefully enough for the patient, in part because he doubted his own instinct. For him, integrating that mistake meant not only gaining an understanding of his own imperfections but also developing a new understanding of his own empowerment.

It's made me more willing to stand up and cut against the grain a little bit, more willing to be the one to say the emperor has no clothes.

Wrestling with the Big Questions

For many of the patients and the physicians, the experience of adversity moved them to ask some of the very deepest questions about themselves, probing the meaning of their existence and their place in the world. To do this they had to open up, to allow themselves to be broken open, and to ask themselves those deeper questions. In order to integrate this experience, they had to be able to put it into a much larger context, to see the bigger picture and define their place in it. Thus, the changes that occurred had implications in many parts of their lives. Dr. C notes that the task of forgiving herself for the mistake she had made was not something that she could accomplish on her own, but in the end was an experience of grace, an experience that then opened her up to passing that on to others and connected her to her patients in a new way.

> Grace. I don't think we could do that ourselves. I think that is the gift of grace. And I think we have to receive it. I think it's always there for us when we're upset and our mind is clouded, but I don't think we're open to receive it. And after reflecting and praying and talking about it, I finally realized that I am also a beloved child of God, just as he was, and that we're flawed by definition, and that we all need grace.

Dr. E reflects on a situation in which he failed to recognize how sick a child was until it was too late. Fifteen years later, he still gets tearful talking about it. The experience caused him to reflect on who he is at the deepest level.

> The humility I gained was not just in the professional domain. It was deep down to my core. I used to try to separate the professional from the personal. I don't try to do that anymore. I'm a physician— that's a big part of who I am. I think these situations are really where we become who we are. When we are faced with a mistake or a situation where we need to forgive or we need to be forgiven, how we handle that says everything about the next part of the road that we are going to be traveling and how we are going to be traveling it—whether or not we are going to be able to move on. If we can't

forgive someone else or if we are not feeling forgiven ourselves, it is very difficult to move on in life in relationships and to be life-giving in a relationship. It's a difficult thing, but I think adversity teaches us hope.

Many of the patients described how their experience of coping with pain caused them to develop a deeper understanding of themselves and allowed them to learn and grow in ways that went far beyond the specific experience of dealing with pain. Some found it hard to describe the changes because they were so profound. Lauren, who had debilitating migraines for years, stated,

I just know that it changed me somehow, but it's hard for me to step back and look at it objectively because it's just integrated in my life so much. But it's made me think differently about life and being alive.

Mary put it this way:

I feel integrated in the sense that you do go deeper in yourself. It's part of character creation. I've become more understanding as I've gotten older, which is really a surprise to me because I used to have such a superficial view of many things that were happening, rather than looking deeper into the situation.

A deep learning occurred in the context of coping with their pain when patients were willing to open up, step into their experience, and to go deep. Tracey offers her perspective:

In my experience, there is something deeper at work and huge life lessons to be learned. If a patient remains in a victim mind-set, those deeper lessons are likely to be missed.

So how do people achieve this kind of integration after a traumatic event? What process do they go through to rework their narrative?

"Working" the Story

If what Calhoun, Tedeschi, and their colleagues have outlined is true, then integration of this event into a new life story happens through an iterative process of what might be called *positive rumination*. That is, through a process of sharing the story, accumulating new experiences, perhaps testing out new ways of looking at things, and finding or creating meaning, this event is integrated into a reworked story that has expanded or shifted to include this experience and its implications. So how did it work for our study participants?

Talking or Writing about It

First, it appears that speaking or writing about the story is one way that people begin to get a handle on how to put things back together in a new way. In the interviews, we noticed that, for many people, simply telling the story of their trauma had a notable positive effect on their understanding of the experience. In some cases the integration seemed to occur during the interview itself. Some of the physician participants had not told their story to anyone before talking about it in our interview. The narrative had become a "silent narrative" that was locked away, with no opportunity for integration. Some of the participants thanked us for the opportunity to tell their story, noting, at times, "I never thought about that until now," or "Wow, I didn't make that connection until right now." A few of the participants emailed us afterward, explaining how much they had gained from the experience of telling the story and reflecting on how it had affected them. When asked what had made it more difficult, most of the physicians said that not being able to talk about it made the experience much more difficult for them.

Dr. T is the ob-gyn introduced in chapter 5 whose patient had a bad outcome that likely could not have been prevented. As many doctors do, she still felt somehow responsible, even though her colleagues tried to reassure her that there was nothing she could have done to bring about a better outcome. The patient eventually sued, and it was one of the most difficult experiences of Dr. T's career. She reflects now with a measure of disbelief about how she told no one, not even her husband, about what had happened.

> I didn't tell my husband about the lawsuit. I just felt like it wasn't fair to put him through all this. So I just pretended that nothing was going on. But I'm pretty transparent. Emotionally, I felt so isolated. He's always been my number one support person. Finally, he just said, "What in the hell is wrong with you? Why aren't you sleeping? Why don't you want to do anything?" So he finally found out, and he was actually relieved that it was just [the lawsuit]. Then he became pretty helpful. Even though I told him not to tell anybody, because I just felt worthless, he told one of my best friends. He's just an amazing human being. With a lot of his help, he made me come to grips with it.

One positive effect of sharing the story seems to be that people don't feel so alone, recognizing that others have been in similar circumstances and have gone on to have full and meaningful lives. Realizing that there are good doctors who have made mistakes means that it is possible to have made such a mistake and still be a good doctor. Consider, for example, Dr. F, who in retrospect perhaps could not have prevented the death of a patient she was close to, but still felt a mix of guilt and grief many years after his death. Years later she experienced a turning point in her coping with the event when she was finally able to share with colleagues in a supportive environment not just the facts of the story, but all the feelings related to it that she had been carrying around all those years.

> I think the turning point for me was when we each shared our story. That was the most emotionally fraught experience. I didn't share

just a story, I shared the feelings. The feelings just came out—all the regret and the loss.

Another positive effect of sharing the story is what people discover, or rediscover, about themselves that helps them to integrate the experience into their life. Dr. X related how helpful it was to talk with a nurse about a missed diagnosis. The nurse did not sweep away her concern or try to reassure her that it was not a mistake. She accepted the fact that it was an error, and then went on to say that it didn't change how she thought about the physician—her capabilities or her goodness. This allowed Dr. X to integrate this error in the context of the other things she knew about herself—that she was a good doctor, generally careful and thoughtful, with an excellent track record. She could learn from this without calling into question everything she thought about herself up to that point.

When she heard me say, "I made a mistake," she accepted that. And then, it was just, "Okay, so what are you going to do about it? What do you feel about it?" So that put it in full perspective—that you can do something wrong and you can tell somebody and get that confirmed but also get confirmed that this is in the context of an honorable or whatever clinical track record and that they're both true. That even somebody who has a good track record can make a mistake. You don't have to say, "Well, you couldn't possibly have made a mistake because you're so good," which is not a helpful thing to say. Or "You made a mistake, so maybe you're not as good as I thought you were." That was useful and that is what I needed to hear, because you can't practice if you don't trust yourself. And you can't practice by completely defining how you practice by avoiding one particular mistake that you made because then you'll do harm in some other way. So there was just some confirmation that I don't have to completely rethink everything. I can assimilate this. That's what was helpful about that conversation.

Reflecting on Positive Changes

Finally, in sharing the story people begin to make some sense of their experience, which helps them integrate it fully into their lives. They begin to see changes that will bring meaning to the experience, and the questions that people reflect on can make a big difference. Having the opportunity to reflect on how this has changed them *for the better* can help them integrate the experience more fully. One physician spoke after the study interview about how helpful it had been to be asked whether the experience had changed her in a positive way. (Many physicians and patients reacted in this way to the positive question.) Being able to reflect on that specific question helped her see that positive changes had taken place and how, having thought about it in that light, she was able to see how her experience of an error meshes with other experiences in her life that together have had a profoundly positive influence. That insight itself redoubled her commitment to continuing those positive changes and applying them to other parts of her life.

Robert Neimeyer describes it this way: "The recounting of traumatic life narratives to others solicits validation of one's experience and provision of social support, both of which can facilitate healing and growth. Indeed, a good deal of psychological research demonstrates the importance of confiding or 'account making' in integrating and transcending difficult life experiences" (2006, 70).

Gaining New Experience and Testing Things Out

For some, gaining new experience by exploring and testing things out is a way to begin to integrate. Once the pain patients step into the reality of their situation, they begin to explore ways that they can take hold of their experience and try out ways of coping that slowly, iteratively begin to shed the cloak of the dominant narrative of being a pain patient. By exploring things like being in nature, meditation, energy healing, prayer, and attention to others, each of them begins to have experiences of themselves other than as a pain patient. These experiences build on themselves, and slowly they start to construct a view of themselves that incorporates, but is not dominated, by the pain.

Creating Meaning through Positive Action

Some people are able to integrate this experience into a new narrative by creating meaning from the event through their own positive action, and that meaning allows them finally to put the event into a context of their life with which they are comfortable. Some of the most stunning and powerful positive changes in our world have come as a result of tragedy that spurred courageous people to create meaning out of that tragedy through positive action.

The Josie King Foundation, for example, is an organization that promotes patient safety. Josie was a child who died as a result of a medical error. Her parents, in partnership with her doctors, came together to create an organization that promotes safer health care across the country. In this positive response to their tragedy, Josie's parents have helped save countless lives. Many, if not most, of our charitable foundations that fight cancer, MS, ALS, and other devastating diseases have been founded out of similar circumstances—suffering and loss that give rise to powerful, purposeful action. That positive action gives meaning to the tragedy and loss and allows people to move forward with a new narrative for their lives that incorporates the tragedy but in the context of this new purpose.

Sue has developed a commitment to helping children and families in developing countries who live in the extraordinarily difficult circumstance of the city dump. She connects her experience with chronic pain and suffering with her commitment to working with these children.

> There are all these families who literally live in the dump. By tending to burns and cuts on their feet, I can contribute when I'm there. Then, back here, I help to raise money for the school that works with the kids who live in the dump. I let my students know about it. So I have a deeper appreciation for the fact that at least I have an option to heal and get well. Some of these kids have nothing, and I can do something about it. I can do what I can for other people in other places, to the extent that I can, and if I can grow as a result of it a little bit, that's great.

Integrating the traumatic event is a crucial step in creating a new narrative for one's life after the trauma. But this is not a onetime thing. Integration is most often an iterative process that takes place over time as the new narrative is being written. As people piece together ways in which trauma has changed them, they begin to explore what their new story looks like and how this new understanding of themselves and their world can play out in their unfolding future. At that point, they begin to write a new story for their lives.

7. New Narrative

YES
Burden and blessing—
two blossoms
on the same branch.

To be so lost
in this radiant wilderness.
—GREGORY ORR

WE TELL stories about ourselves all the time. When I tell my husband about something exciting or interesting that happened to me at work during the day, I'm telling a story about myself. When a father tells his children about what things were like when he was their age, he's sharing a story about himself. We tell stories about ourselves during job interviews and faculty reviews and at social gatherings of all kinds. What may not be as obvious is that we also tell ourselves stories about ourselves. The ongoing thought process that engages us during our waking hours is all about shaping our personal narrative. We go through life shaping and reshaping the story of who we are, why we are that way, and who we will become, and our story is stitched from the many threads of experience and reflection that we encounter along the way. Our personal narratives are like tapestries, and most of the time the threads become seamlessly woven into the overall fabric of our stories. If someone tells me today that he admires the way I parent my child, I weave a tiny thread into my narrative that says, "I am a good mother." A child who experiences an act of kindness may weave "The world is good" into her personal narrative. This process is so rich and exciting that it is rather humbling to realize that the tiniest of events can have a permanent impact on someone's life, once it's woven into their "This is who I am" story. But what happens to the story when trauma or tragedy strikes?

Robert Neimeyer writes that people who have suffered trauma can have their life stories "massively rewritten" (2006, 68) by these traumatic events. He describes a pervasive human "predilection toward 'storying' experience" (69) that allows people to organize and make sense of their own lives. This process of successfully massaging and reshaping our own story, described in the previous chapter, results in a new way of being—of being able to use the pain and suffering in a way that expands our sense of who we are and who we can become. In our study, we came to envision this as a process of adopting a new narrative about the trauma and about ourselves with the trauma fully integrated into our life stories. A significant transformation occurs when we come out on the other side of the struggle to integrate a terrible event into a new understanding of ourselves.

This book began with a question. We have all witnessed remarkable individuals who have faced adversity and been changed in a positive way, and we wondered, *How do they do it? What does this change look like?* In our study and elsewhere, change often looks like a shift toward strength and empowerment, an increased awareness of the world, a renewed appreciation for life, a more positive outlook and attitude, and even a richer sense of meaning about life and our place in the world. We notice this transformation, this creation of a new narrative, when someone who has suffered says, "This experience taught me so much" or "This has changed me for the better." This ability to reframe and integrate a tragedy or trauma stands out as one of the most remarkable aspects of coping with adversity.

REFRAMING

Creating a new narrative is a process of seeing the positive changes that have occurred or could occur from an experience and then weaving those changes into our new story. Many individuals who grow as a result of adversity use a technique called *reframing*. Think of reframing as looking at the same situation or circumstance through a new lens or frame. The situation hasn't changed, but the person viewing it has readjusted her way of seeing, often changing the view 180 degrees.

Matthew Sanford was thirteen years old when a car accident killed his father and his sister and left him with devastating injuries: he was paralyzed from the waist down. He eventually became one of the world's foremost experts on adaptive yoga, teaching the disabled—many of them paraplegics like himself—how to connect with their bodies in a profound way. Asked by an interviewer if he sees himself as disabled, Matthew answers that sometimes he forgets, that he is surprised by his shadow in his wheelchair. "But at the same time, I definitely am disabled. But my life force isn't completely determined by the ability to flex muscles. . . . There's something here—I don't know what it is and I don't care if it's neurophysiologically explained, but there's a presence here that flows through that isn't solely determined by the fact if I can stand up or not" (Tippett 2010). In those early years after his accident, when Matthew was asked, "How did you cope with all this?" he would answer, "Well, I've had two lives. I had one end at thirteen, my life as a walking person ended at thirteen, and I've had this second life, so I'm actually kind of getting *two* lives." Sanford calls this his "healing story," which allowed him to put away "the childhood love of my body" and confront his new reality. We would also consider this version of his story a powerful example of reframing a situation, or seeing the same view with a different lens.

Sam, the mosaic artist we met in chapter 4, eventually was able to reframe his pain, too.

Pain is with you for a reason. Pain is with you to tell your body and your mind, and even your soul, that it needs to heal itself. That's the reason why it's there—to tell your body. It's not there because it's trying to hurt you. It's there because it's really helping you. [Before that] I was feeling more like a victim, rather than allowing the pain to help me to experience the healing process of it.

In his filmed interview, Maurice, a former soldier who likes to iron, was asked to give a title to his story of living with chronic back pain. The title he chose was "Pain Is My Friend." At another point in the interview, he talked about how he has chosen to view his pain. "It's changed my whole viewpoint on life. It can be empowering, or it can be something that imprisons you. You just have to decide what it's going to be. That's how I look at it." In other words, pain can be the enemy, or as Maurice has chosen, it can be your friend.

Emily has lived with back pain for nine years, and her doctor helped her with this reframing technique, directing her to see and react to her pain in a new way.

One of the things that was most useful to me was something that a doctor recommended to me. It was a type of cognitive-behavioral therapy in which we look at how we're reacting to some sort of a stimulus. In my case it was pain, and the way we're reacting to it directly relates to how we're feeling and thinking at the time. Instead of getting angry and saying, "Aw, I don't deserve this—this shouldn't happen to anybody," and then getting frustrated and more annoyed, I'll just take a look at it from a different perspective and say, "Well, okay, it's a fact that it's something I have. There's no choice. I have to live with it. I'm not the only one—there are other people living with it. I'd prefer if it wasn't this way, but it is, so I just have to do the best that I can." By restructuring my thinking like that, it actually has the effect of lessening the way I feel about it, whether it's physical or psychological pain. As for this physical pain, it's still there, but I don't have to react to it. I don't have to feel pity for myself or pretend to be more disabled or whatever. I just do the best that I can and accept it. It's a reality.

In *Choosing Wisdom*, Tracey DeGregory talks about how reframing enabled her to shift from being a victim to being in control. She says,

One way I can look at it is to say, "My body is a mess." Or, alternatively, "My body actually knows more than I do. It knows something is wrong, and I need to pay attention to this." One way is empowering. The other leaves me feeling like a victim. By working with a healer, I was able to start identifying different beliefs. Is this belief helping me? Or is it detrimental? We have a choice about what we believe. By bringing the beliefs out in the open we can challenge them and identify beliefs that are more helpful. We can reframe anything, including our beliefs.

Reframing can thus set the stage for creating a new narrative for our lives. An important point to emphasize when talking about creating new narratives is Tedeschi and Calhoun's notion that posttraumatic growth is about *change*. It "goes beyond resilience, sense of coherence, optimism, and hardiness" (Tedeschi and Calhoun 2004, 4) and is not simply a return to baseline or the way things were before the traumatic event. Growth through adversity is about positive transformation and improvement—changes not in how we feel but in the way we move through the world and interact with others (4). In this chapter, we look at physicians, patients, and others who have integrated their experience of trauma into their understanding of themselves and woven a new narrative for themselves—one that is more expansive, allowing them to move forward with integrity, acknowledging changes in their priorities, and applying the lessons they learned from their experiences.

Changes on the Inside: New Ways of Thinking and Feeling

Sometimes the changes that people make (the new narratives they are writing) are primarily internal changes—changes in the way they think and feel about things, changes in the way they see themselves and their capacities.

Martin Seligman has often been referred to as the father of positive psychology. In his latest book, *Flourish*, he tells the story of Brigadier General Rhonda Cornum, holding her up as the "poster child for posttraumatic growth" (2001, 160). In 1991 Cornum, a flight surgeon and major in the U.S. Army, was on a rescue mission in Iraq when her

Blackhawk helicopter was shot down over the desert. She and one of the surviving soldiers were taken prisoner. She points to several ways that the experience changed her perception of herself and the way she now navigates the world. One of those ways is with an increased sense of personal strength. "I felt far better equipped to be a leader and commander. That is the standard by which other experiences are now measured, so I feel much less anxiety or fear when faced with challenges" (160). Cornum endured something that is unimaginable to most of us, yet she emerged with a surety and strength that can only come with experiencing such a traumatic event.

Darci suffered from severe arthritis and acknowledged that she had a tendency to feel sorry for herself, and not just about her health. Self-pity was part of her personal narrative, whether it was about her work or her life circumstances. But in coping with her pain, she discovered that the suffering had made her stronger and more appreciative of her life and the things around her. Feeling sorry for herself was no longer part of her narrative:

> You can get through anything, as long as you have the will and you've got faith and you've got people who love you. This may sound funny, but I think this pain gave me the best life that I've ever had. I'm not as active as I used to be, but the things I do, I enjoy more. I think, in a sense, my pain was sort of a blessing.

Sam, the artist, woke up one morning with excruciating, shooting pain in both his hands. He was unable to paint or even hold a fork to eat, and he struggled with depression as his pain worsened. He felt abandoned by his friends and came close to being evicted from his apartment. Learning to cope with his pain and his depression changed him by giving him the knowledge that he could prevail in any situation.

> What it does is, when you're in the lowest of lows, you know that no matter what you're confronted with, you'll be able to overcome. Learning to cope with the pain changed me as a person. Let's say

that I'm facing a crucial decision or I'm expecting bad news. It helps me to deal with a crisis because I feel that I'm more able to take control in that immediate crisis environment. It's made me a lot stronger.

Recall our discussion in chapter 6 of the type of narrative disruption that can occur with trauma, where the trauma becomes the dominant narrative. The pain patients described how their lives became dominated by their pain, and their self-concept became engulfed by being a pain patient. In this victim narrative the patients felt helpless and stripped of personal power. Moving forward to live out a new kind of narrative, one no longer defined by pain, was not easy, requiring a continuous change in mind-set reinforced by others. Harriet is a middle-aged woman who was the teenage driver in a car accident that caused the death of a friend. She has struggled for years with severe emotional pain from that event, as well as physical pain from her injuries. After many years of work she has been able to move through this pain to a place of increased compassion and an ability to connect with others. We asked her whether she had any practical advice to share with others living with pain.

The first thing that pops into my head is don't concentrate on the pain. Concentrate on your life because you are not your pain. That is just a component, but there are a whole lot of other things out there that you can do despite the fact that you are in pain. I find that even though the pain doesn't leave, it is still there, that there are times when I could ignore it and concentrate on other things, when I get lost in other things. It doesn't leave, but I can live.

Tim, the law enforcement officer who injured his back, decided after years of struggling with the pain that he didn't want his life to be defined in that fashion anymore, and he began to take steps to move away from a victim mentality. Then he began to feel better. But in creating a new narrative for his life, he found lots of changes that had to be made so that he could live out a different story, one not defined by his pain. He gives some examples of the kinds of changes he made:

> When I call my mother, right away she goes, "How are you feeling?" I had to work with her to get her not to do that, because I don't want the first response to me to be about how I am feeling. I don't want my identity, my consciousness, to be wrapped around what is going on in my body at any given moment.

Making a mistake and harming a patient heighten a doctor's sense of vulnerability. But working through that fear and sense of uncertainty also often results in a discovery of newfound strength in the physicians we studied. Dr. B "doesn't like controversy and likes to talk to people who agree with me." But his experience of an error has strengthened his ability to stand up to those in authority when the situation calls for it. "Now I am willing to tolerate that discomfort, so it changed me. It's uncomfortable for me—that's the way I'm built—but I am willing and able to tolerate the discomfort of the disagreement when it is the right thing to do."

Dr. Q had a similar experience. He said, "It made me a resident who was certainly more willing to speak out about when things were not safe. Yeah. It definitely changed that." And Dr. J's experience of losing a patient on the operating table was so disturbing that she was unable to function for months. Recovery has been slow and difficult, but she looks back on that experience and acknowledges that she is stronger for it. "Not that I would go looking for one of those outcomes. I would not wish that on anybody, but no, I think I would have the wherewithal to work through it."

Having coped with his experience by sharing with others and experiencing "the power of their compassion," Dr. H knows firsthand how important it is to reach out to others in need. And he says that doesn't just apply to medical situations or medical professionals. "I think that if you have had the rug pulled out from under you—which is the way I describe it when things are just spiraling out of control—and you can't do anything about it, that sense of despair is universal." He doesn't presume to know how friends facing difficulties are feeling, but he is able to ask, "How are you doing with that?" He appreciates that talking about it may take time, and that early on he couldn't talk about it himself. "I'm not afraid to keep asking people, 'How are you doing with that?' but I also give them space and respect that. But I try to let them know how healing sharing can be. You're not alone." And like many of the physicians we interviewed, Dr. H's increased empathy extends beyond the walls of his hospital. With friends and family, "I'm also getting better at finding that balance between giving people space but also letting them know that I'm available and willing to listen."

Sanford explains that he was able to craft his narrative through the experience of yoga, and that yoga continues to help him heal his mind-body relationship. This process occurs "as I practice yoga and pay attention and am in love with the world; actually, it continues to heal. Before I started yoga, I really did feel like a floating upper torso." He concludes that now he lives and speaks with his whole body "and that presence was not realized in me before I started yoga."

Sanford has been able to expand this lesson of yoga to the body's aging and its other forms of decay and failure. Now he is able to see that when he was in the accident, his body strove to continue living, and that we have an opportunity to reframe how we approach aging and the physical changes that accompany it. "Your body, for as long as it possibly can, will be faithful to living. That's what it does." He is able to articulate how the body weaves its damaged parts into a stronger whole. "There's a thing in yoga—it's called *pranayama*. It's yogic breathing. And you breathe in a yoga pose for the spaces—I believe this—for the spaces that you can't feel. When you do, your balance increases, your strength increases, your flexibility increases." His compassion for his body extends to others, and through that compassion he has been transformed. "My body does not heal as well as it used to when I was thirteen. That's true. But because of the compassion I can feel for my body and for others, something else is healing."

Sam is certain that his pain has increased his capacity for compassion, particularly toward people who are suffering as he has.

I've also changed by becoming more compassionate to people, particularly toward people with carpel tunnel syndrome. We can all be a little bit more proactive in helping others. I would do whatever I need to do if the opportunity were to arise to help other people who are in pain.

CHANGES ON THE OUTSIDE: DOING THINGS DIFFERENTLY

Through an iterative process of weaving and unweaving the story, a traumatic event eventually can become a rich thread in our understanding of ourselves, becoming part of the larger fabric of who we are in the world. We can take the lessons learned through suffering and apply them in ways that can change how we do our work, how we are as parents, and how we function as community members. Our new narrative can be subtly different or a dramatic turnaround. A colleague, Carolyn, who was diagnosed with breast cancer, once said that the experience of illness changed her in profound ways, and that the transformation occurred through a process of reflection, trial and error, journal writing, and talking a lot with her husband and girlfriends. One of the first things that she and her husband realized was that their children would take cues from them about how to cope with her illness. "In other words, if we were calm, they would be more likely to be calm. If we were frightened, they were more likely to be frightened." It went beyond what they said to their children; it was a more powerful sense of what they conveyed to them through both words and actions. To convey something as important and often as elusive as calm, they needed to work on actually being calm. This realization, this link between her own feelings and behavior and her children's happiness, was her guiding force about how to behave with her children throughout her illness and treatment. When cancer was mostly behind them and life returned to normal, Carolyn realized that she had integrated that lesson into all aspects of her parenting. When her son failed two history tests in a row, she projected confidence in his ability to regain his footing, and eventually he did.

> Of course I don't really wish I'd had cancer. But I'm so grateful that it's made me a much better parent, hopefully a better person. The benefit overall for my kids and my family is pretty profound. I'm not sure how long it would have taken me to figure out this lesson on my own!

Sometimes, like Carolyn and her new parenting skills, a lesson learned as a way to cope with a crisis or tragedy can be applied to other aspects of life. Lessons can be applied in an intentional way; decisions can be made differently than they had been made in the past. Cornum, the army doctor, brought her experience in Iraq to bear on how she cares for her patients. "I felt much better prepared to be a military physician and surgeon than previously. The concerns of my patients were no longer academic" (Seligman 2011, 160).

CHANGING OUR WORK

The experience of a significant mistake among physicians results in a new or heightened awareness of vulnerability, imperfection, and the limits of what we can know. Being doctors with this heightened awareness means making changes in the way they practice that take into account these acknowledged limitations. Such changes are very different from what is typically referred to as "defensive medicine" (for example, ordering lots of tests that are unwarranted just to cover yourself). These are also different from the changes that physicians make in their practice that address the one mistake—for example, always ordering an X-ray after they place a central venous catheter to ensure good placement. The positive changes that we're talking about here are more global and more enduring changes that improve patient care overall and signal a change in the narrative of who they are as doctors.

We are talking about things like emphasizing good clinical teamwork, creating a careful discipline of how they arrive at a particular diagnosis, being aware of the risks associated with doing something that is outside standard procedure, making sure that systems are in place to catch common mistakes, and creating a culture in their work environment that is collaborative, where people speak up if something doesn't look right. These kinds of changes affect everything that they do and are a new narrative for their doctoring.

Dr. M's patient died after a liver transplant, from a mistake that potentially could have been prevented through better teamwork and a culture where people speak up when things seem to be wrong. After that patient's death, Dr. M has changed the way he works:

> We have the opportunity to back each other up when somebody misses something, the ability to acknowledge mistakes and make sure you speak up when you see something, because the right thing to do is get it fixed before it ever goes any further.

Dr. McD is an internal medicine physician who, late one night, had to put in a central venous catheter in order to have vascular access to give urgently needed medications. The routine in such procedures is to check an X-ray after the line is placed, to make sure that it is in the right place and that the lung has not been punctured. The procedure went smoothly, but because of the urgency of the situation and the relative difficulty of getting an X-ray quickly, she made the decision to forgo the X-ray. As it turned out, the line was in the wrong place and the patient had a serious complication as a result. Everything turned out okay, but the physician was shaken. It changed her.

> *A hundred percent of doctors do it this way. You do it this way every other day of the week. Why did you do it differently this time? That's the lecture I gave myself that night and the next morning, and I couldn't even rationalize it in my own head. I still can't rationalize it. So in the future I want to be able to say that I have a reason. There's*

no excuse for not doing something that you absolutely know you
need to do. So that's how it's changed me.

In this case she recognized that, without discipline, physicians can
get sloppy in their thinking and action. Rather than following through
on the standard procedure for the decisions they are making, physicians
mindlessly take actions that, in retrospect, could not be rationalized
and therefore would not have been done had they really thought about
it carefully.

Dr. O is a surgeon who misread a pathology report. The error resulted
in the patient having to undergo another minor surgical procedure. Dr.
O studied carefully why this had happened and made a few changes in
her procedures so that it wouldn't happen again. Now she never calls a
patient on just a verbal report. She also has a cross-check system on all
pathology reports with her nurse. But because the error had helped her
see the reality of her human fallibility, she began to see many opportunities for making her practice safer and has since made numerous
changes to other procedures, including visual cross-checking by the
nurse and physician for labeling and placing the specimen in the con-
tainer, thereby reducing the possibility of mixing up specimens.

Some physicians experienced a shift in values, or a revaluing of
things they had lost sight of before the error.

In the film *Choosing Wisdom*, Dr. Jamie Redgrave talks about how,
after her experience of a medical error and cancer, she vowed that never
again would she allow herself to be in a situation where she did not
spend enough time with patients. She decided that she would take a
cut in salary and schedule longer appointments with patients. She also
found that after these experiences she was more willing to share her
"self" with patients.

Before I felt that there was always a part of myself that I was holding back. Some of it is how we are taught, that we should not share
ourselves, that there is this boundary. But some of my most profound encounters with patients have come because I crossed that

boundary. I have diabetes. So sometimes I say to my patients, "I have diabetes. I take insulin." And that has been really helpful to them.

In weaving her new narrative she has vastly changed how she does her work, and in the process she has rediscovered the joy she felt from that human connection with her patients.

Dr. D, a family physician, experienced profound grief over her delay in diagnosing cancer in a patient she had had a close relationship with for years. In the immediate aftermath and for months afterward, she stayed close to the patient and her family—literally, by going to appointments with her and helping her navigate the health care system. It was a bumpy road for Dr. D. Many times it was difficult to be present, to face the patient and her family, to be reminded of her mistake. But she discovered a certain comfort in staying involved with the patient and being able to help the patient and her family put together the pieces of her medical care. In this process, she rediscovered how much she valued the long-term relationships she had with many of her patients. With all the pressing demands of her job and her life, Dr. D had let this aspect of her professional life, which she enjoyed, slip away. "With all that we do for patients in primary care, when you see somebody you know well with a terrible diagnosis, it's hard when suddenly they're shuttled off and end up in someone else's care—the specialist's. You don't really know what is going on with them, and to me that's a really big hole." She says it feels wrong to tell a patient, "Oh, you've got this terminal disease and now you have to go away, go someplace else."

Dr. D supervises young resident physicians, and "in a two-week period we had six people with new metastatic cancers come in—people who were previously healthy. It was terrible." In that period, she realized, "I felt this real sort of mission to encourage our residents who are caring for these people to stay with them, to stay there and see it to the end." Even if patients go home and aren't going to receive any more treatments, she wants her residents to know that "you just have to stay in touch." Because of her own difficult experience, Dr. D rewove her personal story as a physician and teacher. She has returned to her core values as a physician—maintaining those long-term relationships with patients who are so meaningful to her and her patients, and conveying that bedrock belief about medicine to the young physicians she teaches.

Another physician shared a terrible experience that occurred during his first year of residency training, when he made an error during the delivery of a baby that could have seriously harmed the baby or her mother. They were both all right, but the experience shook the doctor to his core, and he came very close to quitting his medical career before it even started. But the mother forgave him, and the family "didn't reject me, didn't express anger." What he eventually came to understand about that experience was that he had established a good rapport with the mother while she was in labor. "I think I made her comfortable, as comfortable as you can be in labor. And I think that, in time, she kind of got to know me as a person, and she knew I had good intentions and that I wouldn't ever intentionally hurt her."

What this doctor realized was that he would never be able to know everything about medicine. "Because how can you possibly know all you need to know? And I've gotten comfortable with the fact that I don't know." He has learned to look things up when he needs to. He makes sure that his medical decisions are patient centered and that he communicates well with his patients. What it comes down to for him, and this is what he emphasizes to the students who come to his practice, is that "it's all about relationships in primary care." If you make a mistake, and chances are you will, accept it and try to learn from it. "I think that mother was able to forgive me because we had a relationship." This doctor was able to rewrite his personal narrative, incorporating his hard-learned knowledge that he would never be a perfect doctor, but he could be a good, caring doctor.

Some patients and doctors experience a dramatic change in their narrative. Joe was a champion kickboxer who developed chronic pain in his hips and shoulders from many years of training and competition. He was working for a software development company, investing in real estate, and doing very well financially. He lost everything when he began self-medicating with prescription and nonprescription drugs.

In his recovery he started on a spiritual journey that involved a major change in his values and goals.

> In the past when I was holding real estate and had a bunch of rental properties, I think I wanted to play Monopoly and acquire as much as I could. That stuff doesn't matter to me anymore. Now I see the world from a whole different angle. It's more important to develop my soul than to try to conquer the world. I wouldn't trade anything to go back to having the Jaguars and the in-ground pools and all that stuff because the joy that I feel every day is irrespective of how the market is doing or whatever the small stuff is. It's a whole different world that's been presented to me, and the joy from the Lord is just amazing. When you take care of someone else's needs, the Lord takes care of yours.

Some people changed careers or developed a new focus in their career as a result of their experience of adversity. Tracey DeGregory learned a lot about the body's ability to heal itself through her struggle with pain. As she describes it, before her experience with severe debilitating migraines she was not someone who gave much credence to alternative medicine. When someone told her about energy healing, she said, "What in the world is that?" But she went along with her friend's suggestion; at that point she would try anything. The experience was transformative. She found that her understanding of her body's energy was critical in her own healing, and that knowledge eventually changed the course of her life. She decided to dedicate herself to this kind of healing so that she could help others. She became a fully trained energy healer, which has now become her life's work. She has woven a new narrative that looks very different from her pre-pain narrative, one that she could never have predicted.

Like many patient safety experts, Dr. Jo Shapiro became involved in helping physicians cope with mistakes after her own experience. As she relates in the film *Choosing Wisdom*, in the aftermath of her error she had very supportive family members who helped her move positively through this experience. But what about all those people who don't have that resource? How do they get through this? Dr. Shapiro changed her work to devote significant time to developing a peer support program for physicians, sharing her experience and what she has learned so that others don't have to go through what she went through; she also travels the country helping health care institutions develop such programs. She has woven her traumatic experience into a new narrative that is a source of healing for many others.

The individuals in this chapter have successfully managed to change themselves or their way of moving through the world for the better as a direct result of their experience coping with trauma. The disruption in their narratives eventually resulted in new, more expansive narratives. Some have discovered a newfound sense of personal, physical, or even moral strength that grew out of their adversity, but that they now find useful in their daily lives. Some individuals have been able to apply lessons learned about healing, medicine, or coping and used those lessons in multiple realms—in everything from parenting to professional fields. Many have taken the opportunity of adversity to develop a broader sense of compassion toward themselves and others. Some transformed their work or their lives in order to reflect what they learned, their new priorities, their new understanding of themselves, or their newfound capacities. But how do the changes that people report in their journeys through adversity relate to wisdom? Does what people learn and how they change resemble wisdom? The next chapter focuses on this subject.

8. Wisdom

We don't receive wisdom; we must discover it for ourselves after a journey that no one can take for us or spare us. —MARCEL PROUST

C AN ADVERSITY help us discover wisdom in our lives? What do people who have moved positively through difficult circumstances have to tell us about what they have learned and how they have changed?

In the Wisdom in Medicine study, we asked participants to reflect on how their journey through adversity had changed them. What did they learn, and how did they change because of this experience? Did they believe that they had gained wisdom because of this experience, and if so, what did that mean to them? When the participants describe the positive changes that occur in the wake of adversity, they use the language of wisdom. As we see in this chapter, the subjects talk about gaining a greater appreciation of deeper meanings, becoming more open to lifelong learning, having a greater understanding of life's complexity (gaining an awareness that there is not always a right answer), and having more ability to deal with imperfection and uncertainty. They note that they have become more compassionate and more forgiving, and they can see things from many perspectives. They reflect on how they have grown in ways that they could not have, had they not struggled with their difficult circumstances, because their usual way of functioning had to change in order for them to cope.

But the journey in coping with adversity did not really have an endpoint for most people. Instead, it would be more accurate to say that each person developed a direction, and the internal compass was wisdom. Like any direction, we cannot fully arrive at due north, but rather, north becomes a way to travel. No one stayed completely on course, but the participants had a real feel for due north, and their thoughts and actions became self-correcting, based on their deeper understanding of themselves and the world.

Recall from chapter 2 Monika Ardelt's model of wisdom, which has three components: the cognitive, the affective, and the reflective. We use these concepts as touchstones as we consider the subjects' responses to the questions "How did this change you?" and "What did you learn?"

ADVERSITY CAN CHANGE HOW PEOPLE THINK

A Desire to Know . . .

For many people the experience of difficulty seems to trigger a desire to know and to understand as much as possible. For some of the pain patients, that meant specifically understanding as much as they could about their bodies, their minds, how the two interacted, and how they could help themselves. Completely on their own, these successful patients often discovered what helped—by exploring, reading, and being open to suggestions and concepts that they previously might have rejected. They were then able to see how they could apply that openness to learning more globally, and it translated into a deep desire to continue to learn. Mary Anne, who for many years suffered terrible pain from a surgical error, gradually and successfully worked through her pain, a journey of continuous learning. She put it this way:

> I think wisdom is when you never stop learning, when you keep yourself open and you never slam the book shut. That to me feels like wisdom.

Karen is a nurse and an artist. She has lived with pain from fibromyalgia for years, but in her journey with pain has learned much about herself and about her pain, which has empowered her to cope successfully with it.

For me, wisdom is learning about myself, knowing myself, and then being able to research and find things to enhance myself, to make my life better. But it's also sharing what you learn with others, and sometimes seeking opportunities to share those lessons. The human race is so old, and there are so many ancient civilizations that all have something to offer. You have to take it and integrate what works for you.

Learning and understanding were also themes in the physicians' wisdom stories. One of the first productive things that physicians in the study did when faced with a mistake of their own doing was to learn everything they could about that procedure, diagnosis, or illness, in part so that they could understand how they went wrong and, if possible, prevent the mistake from happening again. Some of the physicians did this on their own, because the cases were not discussed openly. But in the ideal circumstance, physicians collectively review cases that don't go well using a process called a *root cause analysis*, or in a morbidity and mortality conference (M&M), discussed in chapter 5. The whole point of this collective review is to discover as much as possible about what went wrong and why, to share that information as a cautionary tale, and to put in motion changes that prevent that situation from recurring. When a doctor or a medical community does this, it tends to perpetuate an openness to learning that builds on itself, and each thing that does not go as well as it could becomes a rich learning experience. Dr. M, who struggled through a very complex situation with a patient and in hindsight realized that he had missed a diagnosis, put it this way:

I don't know what wisdom is except experience that you hopefully turn into an improved experience the next time. I haven't gotten very wise from anything that went right the first time.

The passion for learning triggered by these difficult experiences was quite remarkable. Many of these physicians became experts in a particular field. One emergency room physician, Dr. Z, had an incident where he struggled to get an airway established in a patient. The anesthesiologist (generally the airway expert) who was on this particular night was less experienced than Dr. Z and was unable to help him. Dr. Z's response was to become an airway expert himself.

> After that, I took an airway class and became the airway expert, the go-to guy. I made the department buy a special scope, which I bring to every intubation, and I've never had another bad outcome because I committed to learning all I could after that day. It's just a whole new mind-set.

Becoming an expert can then be taken one step further, as doctors develop a different attitude toward learning than they had prior to the event. In Buddhism this is conceptualized as the *beginner's mind* (Suzuki 2006). Buddhists approach circumstances with an openness to learning and to new ideas that characterizes a beginner, but with the experience of an expert. Dr. O is a seasoned physician who made a simple and common error of misreading a report. That's the kind of mistake that any human-factors engineer will tell you is a typical human error that occurs more often if we are rushed, distracted, or multitasking and happens when we are doing tasks that we've done a hundred times. For Dr. O, that humbling experience made her realize that she always has something to learn.

> I have been getting humble. Because you never want to think that you are hot stuff—that you can't make a mistake, that you can't listen to other possible diagnoses, that you can't learn from other physicians, that you can't learn from the patients and what they are going through. So you need to be humble. And the best doctors— the ones I admire—are willing to learn. They are not easy lessons, but doctors with humility are willing to take these lessons to heart and make adjustments.

. . . and to Understand the Deeper Meaning

This desire to learn also means a desire to go deep, trying to understand the deeper meanings in and for their lives. This deeper meaning helps them not only to make sense of their current circumstance but also to make sense of other aspects of their lives.

The experience of missing a diagnosis was deeply troubling to Dr. I, mostly because she recognized her undeniable vulnerability and instinctively knew that there was really no way to completely protect herself against making a mistake in the future, no matter how hard she tried. This experience is akin to any other experience of human vulnerability—to disease, to accidents, to any kind of misfortune. Dr. H, the pediatric surgeon we first met in chapter 4, realized that this vulnerability connected him more to his patients' experience. It helped him to be more appreciative of life in general and aware of the great gift of being part of patients' lives during their difficult times. He put it this way:

> It made me feel vulnerable. In a way, it's kind of a gift of the profession in that I get to be a part of people's lives at very hard times, and I feel that it continually informs me about what it means to be alive, what it means to be a human being, and what it means to die. In some sense, those traumatic mistakes are part of that ongoing learning process.

A pain patient reported that his pain made him slow down, which gave him the opportunity to be clearer and more observant—to look before he leaps and make better decisions. He sees the deeper meaning of pain for his life as follows:

> Pain slows you down. You can't get wise unless you've got to stop and listen and look and focus—not just glance and holler and bust ass all the time. Wise people are concise. They pinpoint people. They don't move before they know. I am one of those shotgun people.

But if you're in pain, you don't have as much energy to expend. You have to be wiser. It's not that by getting older, people get wiser. It's because they get weaker physically. They have to compensate.

Joe was not a religious man before his pain experience led him down a self-destructive path of self-medication with drugs and alcohol. His life turned around because of his newfound faith. He searches for the deeper meaning in events that happen in his life every day. He finds that meaning in prayer and scripture.

I ask God to please give me his wisdom to understand, because there's so much I don't understand. A lot of his Word is written in parables, so the meaning isn't obvious. You have to think about it, pray about it to get down to what he's really trying to say, and I think there are different levels. Sometimes when I pray a lot about something, then I'll get a new understanding about a certain verse, or someone will teach me something new. That's the kind of wisdom that I'm trying to get at—what God wants me to do with my life.

Lisa, a victim of childhood abuse who suffered from physical defects requiring multiple surgeries, was left with chronic pain that did not abate, no matter what medication she took. She described how her spiritual understanding was the most helpful in dealing with her pain:

I encourage people in pain to find a way of acceptance and peace. I think there are many paths toward that, but they are all moving toward the same thing, like a higher consciousness. I think the spiritual path is more important than the physical to try to cope with chronic pain.

Dr. N is an internal medicine doctor. She made a decision to discontinue a patient's Coumadin (a blood thinner) after the usual period of time following a blood clot in the leg, mistakenly thinking that the patient no longer needed it. But because of an unusual clotting disorder, a fact buried in the patient's medical record from long ago, the patient was supposed to have been kept on lifelong Coumadin. The result was another blood clot. To help her through difficult times, Dr. N described her belief that "love is enough." She put it this way:

> God can't save you from the contingencies and consequences of being human, but love is enough. If you are going to be human, bad things happen, and I don't think God or anybody else has it set in place to keep those bad things from happening. But they can be there to help us though the bad things when they do happen.
>
> The key for me is that I have strong Christian faith. I know that my deepest personal disappointment, my personal error, is when I have fallen below my own standards. I am able to see that and go to God in prayer and say, "Heal me of this. Help me to be the kind of doctor you would want me to be."

Seeing the Bigger Picture

Descriptions of wisdom include the ability to see the larger picture, to understand how this experience fits into the larger picture of our lives, and how we fit into the larger picture of the world. Gaining this wisdom requires some ability to move beyond our singular perspective, beyond the moment, to see how it all fits together in the larger context. As people work through adversity, rewrite their narrative, and explore what that means for their lives, they are able to look backward and forward, situating their experience in the greater narrative of their place in the world. They often have discovered their *growing edge*, the larger life lessons into which they must continue to grow. The bigger picture is really the journey that they are taking. Lisa expressed it this way:

> I think part of it is my understanding that this is not all there is— that I am definitely on a path, and again I do believe that I chose this and it is my responsibility to understand it actually for my good.

Monica developed arthritis as a young adult. She reflects,

> I think of wisdom as more large-perspective—the ability to overlook the trivial things that sometimes in my past took precedence. I think the larger vision predominates now.

For some, this bigger picture is clearly a spiritual or religious journey of discovering the meaning of their lives and their place in the world. Joe's newfound faith was his pathway to recovery. He had been an aggressive young man before his experience of pain brought him to the depths. In his own words, the wisdom he gained and that he continues to seek was "from above" and was focused around his "aggressive" tendencies, which he knows he needs to keep in check:

> James 3:17–18 states, "The wisdom that comes from Heaven is first of all pure. It is also peace-loving, gentle at all times, willing to yield to others." And that's kind of big for me because I was always aggressive. And when I thought of that one yesterday, I was mad because somebody was trying to cut me off in line on the way into the bus, and then I said, "Remember, be willing to yield to others." That's the kind of wisdom I want to have. It just helps me to be a better person.

HUMILITY AND UNDERSTANDING THE LIMITS OF OUR KNOWLEDGE

As we explained in chapter 2, humility figures prominently in most descriptions of wisdom or wise people. Humility involves understanding the limits of knowledge and our own limitations as human beings. Accepting imperfection and the limits of our knowledge and abilities was a major shift in thinking for some of the physicians, and all the physicians struggled with perfectionism. Most doctors are trained to be perfect, and for a good reason. The stakes in medicine are very high, and imperfection has almost unthinkable consequences. People who pursue a career as a physician are usually highly successful students. Many of them have never gotten a B. This high level of achievement and having high standards are all good, but a wise doctor knows that mistakes happen and that perfection is not possible. Patient safety experts know that when doctors are aware of this possibility of error, they are most likely to prevent harm. Openly acknowledging mistakes gives them the best chance to learn how to prevent those mistakes in the future. Physicians who moved through their experiences positively were able to integrate that humility and awareness of imperfection into their understanding of themselves, offering evidence of growing wisdom. As Dr. B put it,

> I'm an imperfect doctor and an imperfect human being, and I can say that and feel okay about it.

Dr. P is an older physician who, in reflecting back on years of experience, felt that failure was critical to young physicians' development and to their ability to handle difficult situations. He was involved in a wrong site surgery early in his career, and speaking of his own failures, he said,

> My error reinforced what I already knew: that I'm not perfect. We're fragile. I've got to be very careful about planning things that are big. I've got to communicate better. I've got to stop myself from jumping to a conclusion. I think that going through an episode like that steels you, in a sense. It makes it a little bit easier to handle stressors in the future because you've been through a bigger stress than that and you know that you can get through one.

Patients also spoke of their experience as teaching them humility. When asked whether her experience with pain has made her a wise person, Lenn, who has been meditating for almost thirty years, put it this way:

> It's a deepening. I feel very different than before. If nothing else, I guess "humility" is the word that I'm looking for. Humility is a word I think a lot of people don't really understand. I think it is one of the most powerful things. It means to feel this enormous gratitude

because you're not taking things for granted. It's not based in the ego, where you say to yourself, *Oh, I'm in control of things. And things are going my way because I make everything happen.* It's as if we can have intentions and we can do things, but then sometimes we find that it's not going our way. And so you have to say, *Now what?* You have to accept that because that's what is, that's what's happening. And you find it gives you these opportunities.

Barbara, a fibromyalgia patient, put it simply, recalling the words of a country-western song:

Sometimes you can't do everything that you want to do and you can't let that bring you down. You have to go with the flow and do the best you can and realize that it is the best you can do. You have to play the hand you're dealt, and there's a song that really has a lot of wisdom. I love this song: "You have to know when to hold 'em, know when to fold 'em, know when to walk away, know when to run." And that's true of life.

Hall uses a brilliant analogy:

In an odd way, humility forms, like a crystal, in the "mother liquor" of limitation. We graduate to a humbled understanding that so much information—about the nature of people and the nature of their interactions, about the foundation of decisions and the pre-diction of future actions and events—remains so inaccessible and therefore so profoundly unknowable that it is only fitting to respond with humility in the face of such uncertainty. (2010, 143)

Tolerating Ambiguity and Understanding the Uncertainty in Life

One of the difficulties for the physicians in our study, like many others in fields in which decisiveness and confidence are necessary, was finding the balance between understanding the ambiguous and uncertain nature of much of what they do and being able to move forward to make decisions and act in critical situations. Medical training fosters the latter, perhaps at the expense of the former.

Experiences of events going wrong bring uncertainty and ambiguity front and center. For some doctors, that meant going through a period where they simply could not function. They could not make decisions in the high-stakes environment when they were so keenly aware of the things that could go wrong, and of the truly ambiguous nature of the decisions required of them. But as the physicians moved through the process of coping with mistakes, they began to achieve that balance and were able to hold these two aspects together.

Dr. I describes her struggle with trying to achieve this balance in the years following her missed diagnosis:

> I've had times where it feels as if, for a few months in a row, I am overly vigilant and other times when the flow is a little better—I am not worrying about it so much. But I think that is part of what I do. You do the best you can to try and head those excessive worries off.

Wisdom researcher John Meacham suggests that this balancing between knowing and not knowing is perhaps a defining characteristic of wisdom. "The essence of wisdom is to hold the attitude that knowledge is fallible and to strive for a balance between knowing and doubting" (Meacham 1990, 181). For a physician this is a delicate balancing act. We learn the facts in medical school, but we learn how that knowledge is fallible through harsh experience. The result can be a paralyzing loss of confidence. Finding our way through to the right balance of doubt and decisiveness is difficult. Meacham suggests that this balance of caution and confidence can be best attained in the context of what he calls a "wisdom atmosphere," one in which there is a supportive network of relationships in which doubts, uncertainties, and questions can be openly expressed and ambiguities and contradictions can be tolerated, all of which can help the person to avoid either over-confidence or paralyzing caution (208). The physicians' experiences with error made them keenly aware of this delicate balance, which is in sharp contrast to how medicine is often portrayed—both to its trainees and to the public—as an exact science, a picture that fails to convey the reality of the ambiguous and uncertain nature of most of what physicians do. Dr. I put it this way:

> We need to recognize how imperfect all of this is. We still do too much of a job telling the public and even students and residents that medicine is an exact science, that if we just do it right, it will all come out right, and that's just not the case. I think I am a lot more tolerant of uncertainty because you realize that you can't fix it all.

Adversity Can Change How People Feel

Monika Ardelt (2003) suggests that the affective component of wisdom has to do with empathy and compassion, which increase as self-centeredness is transcended. Empathy and compassion imply serenity and contentment, because they enable one to accept the possibilities and limitations of life, including physical health and decline.

Increased Compassion

The study participants described how the experience of adversity in their own lives increased their compassion for others who are going through similar circumstances and for others in general, no matter the source of their suffering. The patients found that their experience of pain had enabled them to relate to others with empathy and compassion. But it didn't just give them a way of understanding others; it also cultivated in them a capacity to connect with others, to see opportunities for compassion where they had not done so in the past.

After struggling with pain for years, Karen looked back on that experience and feels that it has given her a way of understanding and connecting with people that she did not have. Sharing her compassion and her experience with others is meaningful to her, as she explains:

It's also sharing what you learn with others, and sometimes seeking out opportunities to share. People tell me I'm the kind of person they could just sit with. They like to be in my company. When they're freaking out, they'll come in, and I've got the music playing, and I've got fresh flowers on my desk, and they say, "Can I just sit in here for a few minutes and relax?" "Yeah, you need a hug?" So I'll give them a hug, and I'll let them just sit and de-stress a little bit.

Monica describes how she has become more open and more compassionate with others because of her own suffering:

I have been able to open up to other people through this because I have a lot more empathy for others and a lot more compassion, and I have more ability to be in touch with others. I think there was a time in my life where I could have gone down a path of isolation and withdrawal, and maybe depression, but for whatever reason, I was able to stay at work and in a community of people. I feel I have good things to share with people who have pain now—various forms. Even if I wasn't doing massage, I feel I still would have a lot of compassion.

Emily tells a story in order to explain how her pain experience has made her different from how she used to be, but also different from some of her friends. Her learning has been about how to treat others, and that has come from an ability to connect with others, regardless of how different they might be from her.

To me, wisdom is knowing how to treat other human beings regardless of who they are, where they come from, what walk of life they come from. I'll give you an example. I invited a male friend of mine to dinner. I'm not a rich person. I said, "Come on. It's on me." So we were walking down the street, and I see this guy sitting in a doorway. For some reason it was almost like the Lord said to me, "Help this person." I reached in my pocket and gave the man a twenty-dollar bill. I would rather have him go eat or whatever, but if that man needed a drink to get him through the night, that's what he needed. And my friend said, "Why would you give him your money? I wouldn't give him my money." I replied, "See that's you, this is me. My father said you never let another human being go hungry. He said if you can't give him money you give him a piece of bread."

Wisdom is simply treating people right. I know that's not wisdom in the sense that most people think, but to me that's wisdom. Wisdom could be having knowledge, having books, knowing how to read them. But to me the best thing about wisdom is to think about how your fellow man is. Maybe if we all did that, this world would be a better place. Treating your fellow man as a human being and decently—that's wisdom to me. Knowing what's right and knowing what's wrong and doing the best you can.

Physicians also described how their experience had given them a greater capacity for relating to patients, and greater compassion for patients who are suffering. Just like the patients, some of our physician subjects also found that sharing their own experiences and their emotions allowed them to connect with patients in a completely different and deeper way.

Up until her experience with a mistake in the operating room, Dr. J had never been able to share her own experiences of difficulty with her patients, even though she understood that her patients may have benefited from seeing someone who was coping well with a circumstance similar to their own. Somehow the experience of her mistake eventually allowed her to be comfortable sharing these other challenges she faced. As Dr. J relates,

With patients I think I have developed a much better sense of compassion and empathy. Where I used to be ashamed or afraid to talk about any personal experience, I have no problems sharing these stories now. That's so helpful to them in helping them come to grips with their situation. That's been incredibly empowering for me.

Similarly, Dr. Jamie Redgrave in the film *Choosing Wisdom* describes how, after coming to terms with her own difficult experiences, she was more willing to be open with her patients. As she puts it, she no longer finds it draining to be with patients in their times of need, because she is able to truly connect with them.

The physicians in the study also reported a greater compassion for other clinicians who had made mistakes and found themselves to be more forgiving and less judgmental of others who make mistakes. Among the physicians' statements were the following:

> There is no prescription out there for the way to do it right. We all just have to do better.

> I'm wiser and I am also more forgiving of everybody else, hopefully myself as well, and that is wise also.

> I am less critical when I hear a story about another physician. And I think I am perhaps a little more sympathetic when bad things do happen.

> I certainly am absolutely more understanding and forgiving of the frailties of others—whether my coworkers or the nurses.

For some, like Dr. Jo Shapiro in the film, this compassion for their fellow caregivers inspired them to become active in trying to change the culture of medicine from blame and silence to openness and learning. Dr. Shapiro has started the Center for Professionalism and Peer Support at the Brigham and Women's Hospital in Boston. This program provides training and support for clinicians at the hospital, preparing them to respond with openness, honesty, and compassion when something goes wrong and supporting clinicians and families in the aftermath. Dr. Shapiro explains,

There's something so special about talking to peers. I think that colleagues can help us forgive ourselves in a way that we have trouble
doing ourselves. And I thought, *We have to harness this!* I mean, this
is so powerful and also so needed. Harnessing the power of community is something I really learned from this experience.

Dr. Shapiro believes that substantial improvement in patient safety
will come when we recognize openly that physicians and nurses, like
other human beings, are vulnerable to making mistakes, and that a
culture of openness and compassion leads to informed and compassionate actions to improve health care.

Adversity Can Change How People See

According to Ardelt (2003), the reflective component of wisdom is a
person's ability to have a clear-sighted perception of reality, decentered
from self, and to consider events from different perspectives. The reflective component of wisdom is the ability to perceive life as it is, rather
than through one's fears and projections. It helps us grow in wisdom
as new life experiences come along. It guards against black-and-white
thinking and mistakes that can occur because we are stuck in one way
of seeing something.

For physicians, this approach is critical to making good diagnostic decisions. Many decision-making errors occur because physicians
remain stuck on one diagnosis and fail to consider all the possibilities
when new information comes in that should lead to rethinking the
initial diagnosis. This error is called *anchoring bias*—and it happens
to all of us—but it is particularly devastating when it happens in the
medical arena. Cultivating the capacity to reflect continuously on decisions and actions helps physicians guard against this potential mistake.
Wise physicians (or wise people), then, are continuously reflecting on
decisions and behavior, taking in new information and questioning,
revising, and improving. They welcome a second opinion and seek

out others' thoughts, particularly from those who might disagree with them, because that helps guard against their own biases.

The Power of Thinking Differently

Physicians and patients alike described an enhanced appreciation for and attention to complexity—the importance of being able to see things from many perspectives and to critically observe their own thought processes. This viewpoint requires a capacity to transcend ourselves, to be able to notice when we are caught up in a narrow way of seeing something and rise above it. Dr. K, a family medicine physician, related a mistake in which she removed the stitches from a wound according to the recommended protocol, but for that particular person and that particular wound it was too soon. The wound broke open, and healing was slow and difficult. In her estimation of the case, she was too reliant on the usual process, so she missed the signs that this particular wound had not yet healed enough for the sutures to be removed.

> That made me very aware of every little thing. What you need to do is to be more aware that there are different presentations and that your goal is healing. I was taught, after ten days, take the stitches out. But not in every case. You have to be a little flexible.

Another family physician, Dr. U, recounted how early on in the diagnosis of a particular patient's presentation she decided what was wrong and treated the patient for an exacerbation of her lung disease. The patient failed to improve, and eventually Dr. U realized that she had made the wrong diagnosis and that the patient was actually in heart failure, a very easy misdiagnosis because the presentations can be quite similar. But in her mind she feels that it took her much too long to consider other diagnoses. Since that experience, she disciplines herself to consider a broader range of possibilities in each case:

Coming out of that, I gained greater appreciation for the subtleties of the diagnostic process. I learned to be real careful about pigeonholing, compartmentalizing, framing people, and dismissing their complaints.

Considering a broader range of possibilities means actively seeking out others' perspectives. For physicians, that means a new desire to partner closely with patients and other team members. Dr. N, because of her mistake in discontinuing a necessary drug, learned the importance of partnering with patients and other team members. Well-informed patients and a close team whose members know how to speak up can help to correct mistakes before they cause harm. They can act as an important counterbalance, keeping physicians sharp and comprehensive in their thought processes. In Dr. N's words,

I think we do have to partner with the patients and make sure that we empower the patients—and the staff—to ask questions. We have to be open to questioning our colleagues, but we also have to be open to our colleagues questioning us.

Dr. N tells of a situation in which a nurse had suggested a course of action that was different than the physician had chosen to take. In hindsight the nurse had it right, but their communication during the case had hindered their collaboration for the best outcome for the patient. The physician took away from that experience a whole different appreciation for the importance of a true team:

Up until that point, I had never really appreciated how, by working together, we can help fix each others' failing a little bit at a time.

Seeing Pain Differently

Some patients who gained the ability to see things from other perspectives began to view their pain differently, which became the building block of their empowerment. Carol, who suffered with pain for years, didn't want her son to grow up with a world dominated by "his mom's pain." That perspective motivated her:

> Chronic pain is something that allows you to look at problems from a perspective that is unavailable to you until you've had certain experiences.

Lauren, who had debilitating migraines for years, found it very helpful to be able to decenter from herself and get a different perspective:

> It's almost like you can see yourself from both the inside and from the outside, and that's something I never used to be able to do. It's almost like being able to watch yourself as you're doing something.

This process of decentering—being able to see one's own thought process and examine it—frees people up to change their mind-set, and thus their experience. Not only is decentering exemplary of wisdom, it can be a powerful tool in controlling pain. Gabriel, who suffered a neck injury and endured years of debilitating pain describes it this way:

> When you are feeling all this pain, and you're just miserable about it, it feels like nothing's going to make you better. You recognize how you can be in a certain mind frame, and it creates your reality. This reality of suffering and misery that I'm experiencing can be altered if I do the right thing.

Gaining Self-Awareness through Reflection

Of the three components of wisdom, Ardelt believes that the most important is the reflective component, because it gives people the capacity to reflect on their own actions and thoughts and to self-correct, thus allowing them to grow in wisdom as new life experiences come along.

Dr. P described it this way as he was reflecting on teaching young medical students:

I think the element of wisdom that's most important is self-awareness. If you know yourself, that's the most important wisdom that you can have. You can't do much to help other people unless you know yourself.

———

In our study of wisdom out of adversity, we chose specifically to study how people can develop wisdom out of difficult circumstances. It is helpful to study extraordinary exemplars of wisdom, like the Dalai Lama, for example, but it is too easy to think, *Well, I'm not them, so wisdom isn't something that is within my reach.* Our subjects taught us that wisdom can come out of difficulty. We also learned that the journey to wisdom is not easy. In fact, one of the things that people in the study commented on is that just making the journey gave them an increased sense of strength and a sense of empowerment that they could then apply to the next difficult experience.

No doubt about it: This journey is difficult, and one that does not always work out well. But these study participants were able to change in extraordinarily positive ways. Part of our purpose in conducting this study was to try to discover what might make this journey a bit less arduous and more likely to result in positive outcomes. We asked, "What made it easier for you to get through this in a positive way?" People didn't find this question hard to answer. Participants had sage advice for those going through difficult times as well as those trying to help others, which is the subject of part 3.

PART THREE

What Helps: Sage Advice from the Field

Sometimes our light goes out but is blown into flame by another human being. Each of us owes deepest thanks to those who have rekindled this light. —ALBERT EINSTEIN

Believe that there is light at the end of the tunnel. Believe that you might be that light for someone else. —KOBI YAMADA

In the chapters that follow, we share with you words of advice, encouragement, and wisdom from the participants in the Wisdom in Medicine study—statements that emerged when we asked them what had helped them along their journey. Some of this wisdom came the hard way, discovering what would help them only after years of suffering. Some of it they learned from others, gifts that they pass along now to people who might be facing similar challenges. When we asked at the end of the study why our subjects chose to participate, the majority said that they wanted to help others—to share what they had learned so that perhaps others might benefit from their experience.

9. Finding Community

I wonder whether you realize a deep, great fact. That souls, all human souls, are interconnected . . . that we can not only pray for each other but suffer for each other. Nothing is more real than this interconnection—this precious power put by God into the very heart of our infirmities. —FRIEDRICH VON HÜGEL

There is nothing so wise as a circle. —RAINER MARIA RILKE

I F WE COULD point to a constant in the healing process for patients and physicians, sharing, talking, and seeking support in community make up that common vital thread. In the film, *Choosing Wisdom*, Dr. Jo Shapiro talks about how important it is to harness the "power of community" to help each other heal. Deriving comfort from colleagues, family, friends, a house of worship, or a support group was the lifeline for many individuals as they moved from trauma to wisdom. That healing cannot happen alone simply makes sense. As Monika Ardelt explains in the film, "We are social beings. We are not just individuals," despite our American credo of rugged individualism which suggests that we should be able to manage well on our own. Our research underscores that our basic human instinct is to reach out to others to heal ourselves, to find meaning, to help heal others, and to serve. Our communal life might actually be enriched by trauma and the need to heal in the presence of others. Educator and author Parker Palmer talked about this in an interview:

> The deepest sense of community I ever come into with other people or God is at those points where I am able to acknowl-

edge my own failure. When I'm successful and shining, I don't need anyone else. But when the brokenness shines through, people connect in our common humanity. There is a lot of joy in finally being accepted for who you are. The fear most of us have inside of us, especially in church or other groups of well-intentioned people is, "If they knew who I really was they would cast me out into the darkness." (Faces on Faith 2008)

This chapter explores the important role in the healing process of community and sharing with others.

Sharing Stories to Heal

We've written quite a bit in this book about finding meaning as a major component of healing and growth. People ask themselves, *Why did this happen? How can I go on?* Sometimes a traumatic event makes us question our long-held beliefs about ourselves and the world ("I am a good doctor." "I am a healthy person."). In some ways, our journey becomes a matter of *reconstructing* meaning in order to integrate what has happened into our new understanding of the world. Such reconstruction happens when we talk about what has happened to us and tell stories about it. "Narratives of trauma and survival are always important in posttraumatic growth, because the development of these narratives forces survivors to confront questions of meaning and how it can be reconstructed" (Tedeschi and Calhoun 2004, 9). Salick and Auerbach suggest that the process of putting a complex event into a story format simplifies it. "The mind doesn't need to work as hard to bring structure and meaning to it" (as quoted in Pennebaker and Seagal 1999, 1250). In describing his resilience training for soldiers, Martin Seligman writes about the construction of a trauma narrative:

The narrative is guided, with the trauma seen as a fork in the road that enhances the appreciation of paradox. Loss and gain both happen. Grief and gratitude both happen. Vulnerability and strength both happen. The narrative then details what personal strengths were called upon, how some relationships improved, how spiritual life strengthened, how life itself was better appreciated, and what new doors opened. (2011, 162)

In his work on posttraumatic growth, Lawrence Calhoun explains in the film *Choosing Wisdom*, "When you face a very difficult set of circumstances, particularly one that may contain within it the possibility of some degree of embarrassment or humiliation, the worst thing you can do is not talk about it." Sharing by talking is a way to make sense of what has happened to us, to see that we are not the first or only person to experience a particular trauma, and to learn from other people's stories. Health researchers have known for some time that our physical and mental health can improve dramatically once we've had the opportunity to put traumatic or emotional events into words (Pennebaker and Seagal 1999). Our own findings also suggest that keeping silent is a bad idea. Many physicians, either due to shame or legal advice, find themselves unable to talk with anyone about their experience. One general internist, Dr. W, noted that her superior

never said a word . . . Not a single word. And nothing could make you feel more abandoned than that. Sure, don't talk about the case, but wouldn't it have been nice to have heard from the chairman who'd recruited you, saying, "Listen, I heard about that case. I'm really sorry. It's a bad situation. Of course, we can't talk about the medical details, but I want you to know that we think a lot of you and we've got your back." It would have been nice to have heard that.

For some, our research interview was the first lengthy discussion they ever had about the error. For many, the interview revealed raw emotions and prompted tears. The pain of keeping silent was real.

Physicians and patients alike found it helpful to talk about their experience. The specifics and the nature of their revelations varied with the individual or the situation; however, the opportunity to talk to others, to share their story, and to seek and find support was perhaps the most important key to moving forward for almost all the people we studied. Neimeyer's research found this as well, that talking about experiences with others facilitates healing and growth because it provides validation of these experiences ("Yes, what happened to you was difficult!") as well as much-needed social support (Neimeyer 2006).

Calhoun in the film agrees:

> You have to be very careful about who you talk to, but it is good to talk about it with trusted people. And I think, to some extent, growth is more likely when you talk to other people who accept you and don't condemn you. The phrase we use when we are training students for clinical work is, "Listen without trying to solve." The child is dead. The medical error was committed. There's nothing you can do. Seek out other people; tell them the story. They need to be trusted people, and they need to be willing to listen to you. And some people need to tell the story repeatedly. There's a beneficial, therapeutic effect, and in the telling of the story, which often changes from telling to telling, some begin to integrate elements of posttraumatic growth.

We saw this effect as physicians shared their experiences of talking to others, either in one-on-one conversations or in some kind of group setting such as a support group, and the effect this sharing had on moving them toward healing. There are important nuances to this, however. For example, physicians did not find it helpful when others minimized or dismissed the idea that a mistake had been made. Rather, an honest acknowledgment of the mistake was more helpful. In addition, it was very important for them to know that they were not the only ones who had ever made a mistake, so sharing of stories was felt to be very helpful. This support helped physicians integrate their human frailties into their idea of what made for a good doctor, and it enabled them to acknowledge that they were, in fact, good doctors despite what happened.

For many physicians who had committed a medical error, the early healing process included talking to a trusted colleague or mentor, someone who had a firsthand appreciation for the kind of work physicians do and the types of patients they encounter. It likely goes hand in hand with self-forgiveness, but physicians found it very helpful to know that they had done the best they could:

> I spoke to some of my colleagues in clinic to talk about what happened. They said they wouldn't have done things any differently, which helped.

Several physicians deliberately sought to share their stories with people who would not necessarily offer support or warm fuzzies. These doctors went to medical experts, more experienced colleagues, or mentors for their perspective about what had gone wrong and to learn how it could have been prevented. Dr. Q, whose patient died of pancreatic cancer, explains why he invited his patient's surgeon out for coffee:

> It was in part because I needed to tell somebody other than my colleagues, who were excessively supportive, that I had screwed up. They were all saying, "There, there, it's awful. . . ." That's very nice, but I needed to tell somebody who was not going to be protective of me that I had screwed up." The surgeon was helpful because he acknowledged her error and honored it by framing it as a learning opportunity. He also provided perspective and assured her that she "didn't kill this person you loved."

Of additional benefit is the reassurance that, despite the error, colleagues still think the erring physician is a good doctor. One doctor, a resident at the time of her error, said of the colleague from whom she sought counsel, "He was asking me how I was doing, and at one point he says, 'Everybody thinks that you are a good doctor,' and that really helped me. That was so important, because I was still carrying around so much shame and guilt." The colleague also told her that all the other residents were concerned about her, but they were also concerned about themselves, worried that the same thing could happen to them someday:

> Everyone was just thinking, *Oh, my God, that could have been me.* That was powerful, and that was one of my paths to healing. I realized, *Okay, I don't want to quit.*

In the film, Dr. Jamie Redgrave shares another story, the "Pot of Errors," about reassurance and the benefits of knowing that you are not alone. She recounted her experience at a conference she attended where everyone—the older physicians and the younger residents—each wrote a story about an error they'd made. They put their stories into a pot, and each took one out that wasn't their own and read it aloud to the group. Much discussion ensued about how these things happen and what doctors can learn from their mistakes.

> We got to the end of it and I felt like, *I'm not resolved yet.* So I said to everyone, "But wait! I feel like mine was the absolute worst mistake," and everyone was like, "No, mine was the absolute worst." "No, mine was!" I realized that we all still had this sense: we were all holding this weight, this huge weight, this burden. We hadn't let it go yet. When we started to do that—to say, "Mine was worst," "No, mine was," and not even to say what they were, but just to say this is how we felt—then we started to feel better because we realized that we all felt the same way about it.

Sharing and Integrating Emotions

In their studies about narrative and health, James Pennebaker and Janel Seagal have explored why writing and talking have such a powerful impact on health. One explanation, they suggest, is that

the act of converting emotions and images into words
changes the way the person organizes and thinks about the
trauma. Further, part of the distress caused by the trauma lies
not just in the events but in the person's emotional reactions
to them. By integrating thoughts and feelings, the person can
construct more easily a coherent narrative of the experience.
Once formed, the event can now be summarized, stored,
and forgotten more efficiently. (Pennebaker and Seagal 1999,
1248)

We saw a powerful example of this when we offered to a group of health
care providers a three-day workshop on coping with error. On the first
day, we asked all the participants to write about their error experience
and share it with the group. Each of the participants cried while reading
their story, as did the listeners. The emotion was palpable and cathartic.
On the final day, when we asked participants to focus on ways they may
have benefited from the experience and how they might move forward
from here, there were no tears. All the participants were focused and
pragmatic, ready to begin the work of learning and growth. After the
emotional and deeply felt sharing of the physicians' medical error stories, a space suddenly opened up for moving forward and constructing
positive change and healing.

Unfortunately, physicians have many more opportunities to talk
about the technical aspects of a medical error than the emotional
ones. As we saw in chapter 5, morbidity and mortality conferences
are designed to allow doctors to meet privately to determine why a
mistake happened. In the best of circumstances, these conferences
provide information to prevent similar mistakes in the future. Even
when that happens, the individual physician who may have caused
harm to the patient is left struggling to cope with the emotional pain
alone. Physicians talked a lot about pivotal moments when they were
able to speak not just about the medical aspects of what went wrong
but the emotional experience as well. For Dr. H, the pediatric surgeon
whose story we chronicled in part 2, the pivotal moment came in a

physician support group. For Dr. L, that moment came when she shared the emotional side of her error while on a panel of physicians sharing their stories as well as their feelings.

The Schwartz Center for Compassionate Healthcare has taken great strides in creating opportunities for dialogue about the emotional aspects of providing care. This nonprofit organization, based at Massachusetts General Hospital, was founded by Kenneth Schwartz, a health care attorney who died in 1995 at age forty from lung cancer. Throughout the course of his illness, he came to appreciate the profound importance of a touch, a kind word, and other moments of compassion from his caregivers. Before his death, he gave instructions for the creation of the center and its mission to foster compassion in health care. Schwartz Center Rounds, the center's signature program, are now held at two hundred hospitals in thirty-four states. Unlike traditional medical rounds, these hour-long sessions bring together caregivers from multiple disciplines who are directly involved in a difficult case to talk about the emotional side of the experience; many of these cases involved unintended outcomes or errors. Following a panel presentation, audience members share their thoughts and experiences. An evaluation of this program found that providers who attended them felt more supported, less stressed, and less isolated (Lown and Manning 2010).

Support Groups

In the film, Calhoun underscores the importance of social support in recovering from trauma:

> From the point of view of the person who's in the tragic situation, I think a key element is to seek out other people, talk to them, tell them what happened, tell them the story. But they need to be trusted people, and they need to be people who are willing to listen to you.

Support groups offer one opportunity to share stories with trusted people and also to hear others' stories. Ardelt explains their benefit:

One of the reasons why support groups can be really helpful is they provide a way to share experiences. You feel support from other people, you know you are not alone, and that gives you the strength to face it head-on, to be in the present moment, and then to do what needs to be done.

When a support group did not exist when she needed one, Dr. Jo Shapiro decided to create a peer support program at her hospital that continues to this day. She explains,

There's something so special about talking to peers. I think that colleagues have a way of helping us forgive ourselves in a way that we have trouble doing ourselves. I thought, *We have to harness this! This is so powerful and also so needed.* Because one thing that I've come to learn was that I wasn't the only person who has gone through this experience, and I certainly wasn't the only person having those feelings. Though I was lucky to have the degree of support that I did, there are plenty of people who don't. Whether you have family support or not, there's something special about what a colleague listening to you and witnessing with you—your feelings—can do. I decided I wanted to do something with that.

Many patients relied on support systems, formal and informal, to reduce isolation and open themselves up to new relationships; they also learn from each other in these groups. Kathy, who has suffered from migraine headaches since she was a teenager, has found help and comfort from an informal network of chronic pain patients. Although they don't all suffer from migraines, they do share an understanding of what facing daily pain is all about:

We've gotten to know each other. When you have pain, you get to know other people who have it. I've lived here for about eight years, and we've kind of gotten a loose group together. We know each other, even though we don't necessarily travel in the same circles, but we keep each other informed about what is going on in our lives. If we hear about a new procedure, we are in tune with others' problems or pain issues, so we say, "Hey, I was reading this article about such and such, and I thought about you." We are emailing or we are talking or we are doing whatever so we keep that going. It's really important that somebody else understands.

Our research among doctors also found that sharing stories about coping with medical error in a safe environment can be the most powerful antidote to shame and guilt. Sharing opens up new recognition of our better selves as well as a sense of being connected to others who share our experience; we find that we are not alone. The sharing also provides a kind of intimacy with others that we rarely afford ourselves. Rachel Naomi Remen writes in *Kitchen Table Wisdom*:

> At the heart of any real intimacy is a certain vulnerability. It is hard to trust someone with your vulnerability unless you can see in them a matching vulnerability and know that you will not be judged. In some basic way it is our imperfections and even our pain that draws others close to us. (113)

We must be intentional about first creating a space for intimate sharing and then providing an opportunity for constructive writing and reframing, also through narrative.

Finally, a beauty and strength also come from knitting together our narratives, in small group sharing or in reading about or seeing others' stories on film. In the discussion guide to the powerful memoir, *Half a Life*, by Darin Strauss, the author asks a friend if he may share in his book the friend's story about his mother's death. His friend replied,

> It sounds lame to say that hearing *your* story changed my life but it did. Just knowing someone else has gone through something and made it out. And if you put my story in your book, then maybe some other reader will be affected by *that*. And so my mother's story will be in some small way knitted

with that person's story, as well as your story, and my story. And so on. (197)

Writing Instead of Talking

Sometimes a community of supportive listeners is not always available, as we saw with many of the physicians in our study. As Neimeyer writes, "It is worth emphasizing, however, that not all disclosures of personal tragedy will be met with sympathetic, concerned, and helpful responses." This is especially true if the trauma is not socially sanctioned, such as a medical error or an injury caused by a suicide attempt or a drunk-driving accident. The more outside the social norms, "The more unlikely it is that sharing the narrative of one's loss with others will secure the sort of validation and support that fosters integration of and growth from the experience" (Neimeyer 2006, 70–71).

What can we do if, for whatever reason, we do not have access to a support group or trusted friends? Fortunately, there is evidence that writing about the traumatic event can have powerful benefits, similar to those of sharing with others. Writing also provides an opportunity to shape our story, to begin to understand what happened, and in the process to put us back in the driver's seat at a time when we may feel totally out of control. Gregory Orr, poet and author of the memoir *The Blessing*, said about the process of putting difficult experiences down on paper (or the electronic equivalent):

> Before I was powerless and passive in the face of my confusion, but now I am active: the powerful shaper of my experience. I am transforming it into a lucid meaning. (Orr 2006)

Susanne Seuthe-Witz, a sociologist who studies the effect that writing poetry has on cancer patients at the Tumor Biology Center in Freiburg, Germany, believes,

> it is possible that important feelings receive positive expression in this fashion and that patients no longer feel like vic-

tims but creators. The words are like a part of themselves the patients can work with. In this way, they are no longer ruled by their fear but rather rule the fear themselves. (Sautter 2010)

Many of the patients we interviewed wrote in journals, and several doctors did as well. Dr. L, the physician whose friend died as a result of her misdiagnosis, told us that she often wrote stories and poetry, even letters to the patient's family, as part of her healing journey. "In an early draft I write in the second person. So there's a 'you' in the piece. And I realized that it's really just me talking to me."

If a supportive community is not available, writing is. Putting words on paper to craft a narrative of the event or experience has a similar impact as shaping it into a more manageable entity. Even without the support and validation of sharing your story with others, writing can be extremely therapeutic.

Sharing Stories to Help Others

As we see in more detail in chapter 12, helping others is an important aspect of growth and wisdom following adversity. As we talk about community and sharing stories, we need to include the role of stories as a means of helping others or effecting change. Many physicians and patients come to a place where they want to share their experiences so that others can learn from them. They also find satisfaction in lessening someone else's sense of isolation following injury, illness, or a medical error.

When patients or physicians publicly share their story, the potential benefit exists for others coping with similar circumstances. Narratives and the images they convey are the best way to share the richness of the experience (that of physicians or patients who cope positively), and a powerful means of effecting change. These stories—images of successful coping and meaning-making captured in our film and elsewhere—can be powerful tools in helping physicians and chronic pain patients move through adversity toward wisdom. "The narratives of trauma and growth may also have the effect of spreading the lessons to others through vicarious posttraumatic growth. These stories then transcend individuals and can challenge whole societies to initiate beneficial changes (Tedeschi and Calhoun 2004, 9). These stories of success could transform the way that physicians and patients see themselves and their own possibilities. The stories can also reveal to others in the larger society that, with appropriate interventions and support, even people affected by tragedy and pain can heal and become strong. Narratives can influence policy and program development to address the emotional needs of health care providers, patients with chronic pain, and people in any group who have experienced trauma.

By shining a light on these examples, we hold up an ideal image to emulate. Patients often say that having role models for healing is very helpful, and they, in turn, find purpose in serving in this capacity for others. Researchers have observed that people who have experienced trauma actually foster their own growth and healing by feeling useful to others (Salick and Auerbach 2006).

One patient, Sue Holden, spoke about her husband, who had a chronic medical condition that caused flare-ups of severe pain. He had been her "role model for healing":

> Yeah, he's very much that person. And I guess one of the words I didn't use but that I would use is *respect*. But my respect for him for dealing with it and for knowing that—I mean, he had to live with it in a different way than I do. Mine is only going to get better. It's not a disease that can flare. I have great respect for him—the fact that he handles it, that he works through it, that he's as gracious as he is about it. He doesn't take it out on anybody else, ever. He's a pretty great guy. Strong. I feel incredibly lucky to have him here.

Physicians speak often about using their own stories to help others who are facing a medical error or a lawsuit. They also talk about sharing their story to prevent other physicians from making the same mistake.

A few spoke quite publicly about what had happened. Some used their experience to teach young physicians in the classroom. Dr. W, whose patient had died because she had failed to diagnose a heart condition, suffered in isolation for more than twenty years. She had never told anyone her story before the interview, and she hoped that maybe something good could come out of her situation after all.

> This is the first time I've talked to anybody outside of my husband and my attorney about it. I guess I hope that by talking to you— somebody who's trying to use this information to help others— maybe I can help. Because right now it's all locked up inside of me. If what I have to impart could be helpful for others in the future, then I'd like to contribute to that.

This compassion for others, not wanting others to suffer as she did, nourishes the healing process. In chapter 10, we look at compassion and gratitude as important facilitators of growth.

10. Gratitude and Compassion

A loving heart is the truest wisdom. —CHARLES DICKENS

Gratitude is not only the greatest of virtues, but the parent of all the others. —CICERO

THE STORIES TOLD by the physicians and patients often expressed strong feelings of gratitude and compassion. They talked about the ways these positive emotions helped them get through difficult times and how these feelings grew as they moved along the path. Many of the pain patients spoke about consciously cultivating positive feelings. They kept gratitude journals that helped them maintain a positive attitude and sometimes just get through another night of pain. The physicians also took deliberate action that led to emotional resolution and strong positive feelings. Dr. C, who failed to diagnose a case of lung cancer, found it very difficult to ask her patient for forgiveness and afterward felt deep gratitude for her vocation, plus greater tolerance and feelings of kindness. Like many of the people we interviewed, in the end she was very grateful for her struggle. Pain patients who healed after years of pain and determination to get well gained a deeper appreciation for things they had previously taken for granted, including the ability to heal and work again. Many participants said their own suffering helped them feel the suffering of others. They now felt compassion when they once might have felt irritation and chronicled how they were moved to help others make it through difficult circumstances.

Choosing a Positive Path

Leih has lived with chronic pain since infancy and has spent a lot of time thinking about how to live well with pain. At the end of chapter 4, she describes her "bouts with forgiveness" and the cycles of learning that go along with not getting it right the first time. Leih developed her positive attitude during her many childhood hospitalizations. She sees that she has a choice to take a positive or negative path, and that being thankful and "finding the silver linings" helps. When she describes her philosophy about living with pain, she has a disciplined and determined spirit, but she admits that it's not always easy to follow through on her choice to stay positive.

> I started realizing that I can go this way or that way. If I go down this path, I am bitter, I am miserable, I make everybody around me miserable, or I can go down this other path. I said, *I'm going down this path to make the most of everything I can and enjoy every little thing I can and not sweat the little things.* These all sound like clichés and they are easy to spout off, but they're not quite as easy to put into practice. I think pain and other related experiences that cause the pain led to my basic way of approaching life and the world.
>
> One of the things I have learned from dealing with pain, and which I believe many people do come to understand when they go through difficult or life-threatening experiences, is to value everything and anything that is positive in your world and your life. Pain is definitely a happiness drainer. And if you are going to be dealing with pain for any extended period, it only makes sense to work to minimize that happiness drain as much as possible. I will be the first to admit that, sometimes, you really have to reach deep here. Being thankful for having a roof over your head, food on your table, gas in your vehicle, air to breathe, and similar basics may seem rather silly, but I have found it does work. Every thought devoted to a positive idea is one that can't be devoted to a negative idea. And I do believe that most of us have a lot of things to be thankful for, things

for which we can generate feelings of happiness if we only focus on them. The more you do so, the more it decreases the happiness drain. I am a self-proclaimed expert at finding silver linings because there are always positives and benefits that come from everything, whether it is a positive or a negative situation.

Maurice, who was injured while in the armed forces, has lived with back pain for several years. He describes his feelings of compassion and gratitude but also says that sometimes he becomes focused on his own suffering, which limits his perspective. He needs a reminder to "wake up" and remember these feelings:

I've always been compassionate because of my upbringing—just things I've gone through and traveling around various countries and seeing how blessed I am to be born in this country. I think the poorest of the poor here doesn't equal poverty outside America. Sometimes I can be selfish. It's just human nature. Sometimes I can be self-pitying, saying, "Woe is me." Either I slap myself or God slaps me, or somebody else will slap me: "You need to wake up and be thankful."

Leih and Maurice are good examples of the conscious cultivation of well-being that is the hallmark of the positive psychology movement (Seligman 2011). Studies show that cultivating gratitude, optimism, forgiveness, and kindness helps people get through difficult circumstances and live more fulfilling lives. Choosing a positive path is one thing, but it often takes grit and determination to stick with it (Peterson 2004).

Cultivating gratitude is valuable, since practicing even a little bit of it is easy to do and can make a difference in how we feel. In a study called Counting Blessings versus Burdens, one group of students—the blessings group—wrote down five things in the previous week they were grateful for, while the burdens group made a list of five things that irritated or bothered them (Emmons and McCullough 2003). The gratitude lists contained experiences like these: "waking up this morning," "the generosity of friends," "to God for giving me determination," "for wonderful parents," "to the Lord for just another day," and "to the Rolling Stones." Students in the burdens group wrote down "hard to find parking," "messy kitchen no one will clean," "finances depleting quickly," "having a horrible test in health psychology," "stupid people driving," and "doing a favor for a friend who didn't appreciate it." After nine weeks of making a weekly blessings or burdens list, the students in the two groups differed in many measurable ways: The blessings group felt better about life in general, were more optimistic about the coming week, reported fewer physical symptoms, and exercised one and a half hours more per week than the burdens group. In follow-up studies, students were asked to keep daily rather than weekly gratitude journals. Daily cultivation of gratitude led to students being more likely to help someone in need, sleeping better, and improved mood, as well as increased gratitude and optimism for the week ahead.

Cultivating Gratitude

Many of the pain participants kept gratitude journals. As with the students in the psychology experiment, the positive effects of this practice were obvious:

> When I heard about the idea of the gratitude journal, I started keeping one. When you have to think about it, you find out that there is a whole lot to be grateful for and you try not to repeat . . . "I'm grateful for today," "I'm grateful for waking up today." When you don't repeat, then you have to think about the other little things like "I am grateful for chocolate," "I am grateful for the color yellow," "I am grateful for the spring and the flowers." I appreciate that there is a lot to be grateful for. I hear people complaining and when nice things happen to them, they don't see it. I say, "Look, you've got to take your happiness where you can find it." Instead of complaining all the time, look for something good.

Gratitude helps, too—at least I'm alive to see my daughters finish college and grad school. I count five gratitudes in the middle of the night when the pain medicine has worn off and I'm waiting for the new dose to take effect. Try to think of one positive thing to say to someone else. And use the gratitude list—five a night for me.

I learned about a gratitude journal eight or ten years ago. I remember that the first time I picked up that journal, I went blank. What can I say I'm grateful for? I was supposed to write down three things I'm grateful for. Then I got into that habit. Now, if I take out a piece of paper, I can write down so much more than that. I think that's very, very important.

If I had practical advice for anybody, as loopy as it sounds, it would be to count your blessings—every single day. I never let it pass. I spend time going over what I'm grateful for, how much gratitude I have. I'm really grateful. I mean, I have an easy life. I can do what I want to do and manage my pain. I feel like I've been given a second opportunity to reevaluate myself and my life. And I'm grateful for my husband and I'm grateful for my dog.

I would say that I am grateful for all the struggle and pain because I have really learned a huge amount. I have a lot of blessings and things to be grateful for. I can see, I can hear, I can walk, and you look around and there are so many people who can't. I have a home; there's lots of people who don't have a home. So we do have to count our blessings. Sometimes we just have to talk to ourselves and be grateful for what we have.

Carolyn, a colleague of ours who had breast cancer, talked about the positive feelings she gets just by saying "thank you."

> I am very aware of the people and the places in my life that have been good to me. And I know how to say "Thank you," and I know how to give back. When someone is good to me or good to my boys, I go back and say "Thank you." When you do things like that, you get good feelings inside. "Boy, you were special, and boy, you helped me when I needed you—thank you very much. Thank you." It's a good feeling to say "Thank you."

It is easy to understand why the pain participants kept gratitude journals. Counting life's blessings is easy to do and has the power to improve well-being beyond a momentary uplift in mood. It makes sense that many would cultivate this practice to keep up their spirits. It may be surprising, however, that many pain patients felt grateful for their experiences of chronic pain. Many talked about the ways in which living with pain was actually a gift. The unexpected silver linings were the positive feelings they felt after living through the hardest times. Their experiences show that living through suffering and pain can give us a greater appreciation for things we used to take for granted and increase our compassion for others who are suffering.

The Silver Linings of Living with Pain

More Appreciation

Darci was an active and athletic young woman who developed degenerative arthritis in her spine and knees.

> Pain has made me appreciate my life more—the things around me. In a sense, my pain was sort of a blessing. At one time, I took so much for granted. I mean, I could get up; I could go; I could run. I could do whatever I wanted to. So you think, *Oh, this is something you're going to have for the rest of your life.* That's not necessarily so. When it's taken from you and you gradually get it back, it's worth

a lot more than it ever was. That's why I say: the pain in a sense is a blessing because I know I'm still here, I know I'm alive, and I appreciate each day.

Lenn, introduced in chapter 4, talks about her appreciation of pain-free moments.

Consider all the things that you take for granted—your health, your mobility, and just being pain-free—until your mobility is suddenly limited when you're suddenly in pain. After you've experienced extreme pain, every moment that you spend out of pain, you're just so grateful for it. When you're out of pain, you're like, "Oh, wow! Oh, okay. I feel great." It really makes you a lot more grateful for what some people might think are little things. They're not little things. Being pain-free is not a little thing once you've experienced great pain and once you've experienced chronic pain.

Jane is a vibrant seventy-six-year-old woman who took some time to recount all the emotional and physical pain she has lived through. In addition to a son severely injured in an accident, she has had to deal with back injuries and polymyalgia rheumatica, an inflammatory condition that can cause severe muscle pain and fatigue. Despite all these experiences, her feelings of gratitude are strong and clear:

My son was in a very bad automobile accident. I don't know whether it was anger, but something was really hard on me through that. With all the disappointments and the trials that come into your life, I think writing helps, talking with friends helps, being grateful for what you have rather than what you don't have—just that mindfulness. It's a little like prayer, but it's more of a grateful heart.

More Compassion

Lauren has lived with migraine headaches for many years and describes the empathy she feels for others:

It's definitely made me more compassionate to other people in pain. If somebody says he has a headache, I immediately understand what that's all about and I really feel empathy for people. I think my life has changed so much. It's like I can't see it anymore, like a fish doesn't know it's in water.

Even when no solution was in sight, pain also brought positive changes. I expanded my sense of compassion, not only for those in a similar situation, but for anyone who was suffering or struggling.

In the physicians' stories, forgiveness often played a significant part in resolving the emotional burden they felt. The steps they needed to take were often challenging and required some toughness. Forgiving oneself can often take time and can require more persistent inner work than receiving the forgiveness of others. Once achieved, the path is open to strong feelings of gratitude and compassion.

Forgiveness Brings Gratitude and Compassion

It took a lot of courage for Dr. C to ask her patient for forgiveness after a diagnostic error, but in the end she was filled with gratitude at his reaction, and ultimately it brought her many other positive feelings.

It definitely opened my eyes to the awesome privilege that we do have and that I'm in medicine as a calling. To me, it's not a job or a profession; it's a calling. It made me much more awed at the power that physicians have, and to be very respectful of that and not take it for granted. That's probably the biggest change: I appreciate the fact that there is tremendous power to take care of people's health and to see them at their best and their worst in their life, and that it's a gift. I'm a much more grateful person, and I'm a much more tolerant and accepting person—just an overall transformation in my feeling of gratitude and acceptance of power and grateful that my eyes were opened with my patient and that he had a good out-come. Then you develop tolerance of others who make mistakes. I understand that they're not perfect because I know now that I'm not perfect, and I still accept them when they do make mistakes.

After Dr. C's patient forgave her, it took some inner work for her to be able to forgive herself. We hear more about the work she did, the quiet reflection and prayer that helped resolve her feelings of guilt, in chapter 11. In the end, forgiving herself and feeling compassion for her own limitations led to many significant positive changes, including deepened gratitude for her profession, greater empathy for others who make mistakes, a more forgiving attitude toward her students, and greater feelings of kindness.

I used to be pretty hard-core—the students used to call me Dr. Discipline. I used to teach by the Joe Friday method of interviewing. Remember Joe Friday, from *Dragnet*? "Just the facts, ma'am." And the students and residents had better be A+. I had pretty high standards, high expectations. I'm a lot more tolerant and accepting now. Basic human kindness is one of the main things that we can give each other.

Dr. K was just beginning to practice family medicine when a cut she sutured for a patient broke open, became infected, and took many weeks to heal. Her patient was very upset with her because of having to live with the cosmetic issue for that amount of time, although the patient's lack of proper wound care was partly responsible for the wound opening up. Dr. K describes her compassion for his distress:

People have denial initially. Kübler-Ross is right. I've learned that, and that really made me pay attention to those five stages of grief— denial, anger, bargaining, depression, and acceptance.

I think he was in denial about the fact that there might have been other factors. But then it made me think. That was the turning point for me. By acknowledging what your patient is feeling, it made me really realize that no matter what you do in medicine—even if the patient might have done something that caused the problem—you as the physician have to have compassion. Because if that happened to my body, I'd feel the same way. And one of the things in medicine that's really made me try to get better at what I do is understanding that you've got to have compassion. Even if you don't think that the entire mistake was yours, absorb a little bit of that blame, because, after all, you're the doc, and you've got to pay attention to that.

It's a hard field. I just feel that if you can surmount your ego to be more compassionate with your patients, then you're going somewhere with what you set out to do as a physician—to help people. The turning point was not just realizing that now I need to be more careful, but understanding how much more compassionate I need to be and absorb that. It was such a small incident, but it was a really important learning experience for me.

Healing Brings Gratitude and Compassion

Jenny was an active young woman, playing soccer on the weekends and developing her flower, herb, and vegetable farm. But a back injury kept her from these activities for several years. She explored many approaches for healing, including a physical therapy called the Egoscue method and immersing herself in the healing waters of St. Winnifred's shrine in Wales. She describes her experience at the shrine in chapter 13. Jenny nourished the hope that she would get well and eventually made a full recovery. She returned to work and expresses the gratitude she feels in being part of a creative process and sharing her harvest with the people she loves.

Once my body was healed and once the pain went away, I was able to go back into my chosen profession, which is to farm and garden. When the pain was severe I was very disappointed and disgruntled and disheartened that that dream had to be shelved. So I have tremendous feelings of gratitude that I have been able to go back into farming and gardening, which fills me up spiritually, fills me up physically, fills me up communally. There is that extreme gratitude. It has just been a life-changer to go back to my chosen profession of working the land, which for me is a very spiritual experience. For me, working the land and being a part of growing things is a part of communing with the creative force of the universe and is very much about stewarding Mother Earth. Just taking care of the soil, taking care of the plants that are growing from the soil, harvesting them, giving a prayer of gratitude when you are harvesting them, and then sharing them with people in your community and people you love—it's just a full circle for me.

Betsy is a nurse who works in developing countries with disabled children. She was injured in a serious car accident, and her recovery took several years. Like Jenny, she tried many different physical therapies, and she was also successful at getting the insurance company to pay for weekly massages. Betsy and Jenny shared a determination and optimism that they would eventually heal. The gratitude they expressed for the healing process is heartfelt, and according to what we now know about the power of these positive feelings, it likely contributed to their complete recoveries.

It was rainy season when I was in Africa, and I was thrilled when I didn't have to lie flat in my bunk. I could sit up in the chair, in the lounge area, on the weekends—didn't have to lie down now to rest. I could just sit up. I remember just sitting there, watching it rain, and thinking, *It's okay. It's the rainy season. I'm okay here, and I'm actually sitting up.* That was huge. Pain has made me more appreciative of people who are in longer-term recovery and who don't look like they're hurting, but they are. People do hurt. I always say the blessings outweigh the struggles, even though that scale sometimes seems very balanced. It's not. There are more blessings than there are struggles. But when you go through it, just look for the blessings again.

COMPASSION IN ACTION

As a teen, Harriet was driving during a car accident that caused the death of a friend. Many years later she still suffers emotional and physical pain, but her experience has given her compassion that helps her connect with the suffering of others. She relates her experience of seeing a grumpy elderly woman's positive nature that others couldn't see. She quietly ignored the older woman's negative moods, focused on the positive, and helped turn a situation around.

> Pain has certainly made me more sympathetic and more compassionate. There are times when I can see that a person is having a problem and other people can't see it. I remember when I was doing an internship at a senior citizens' home and there was this one woman nobody could get along with, but it turned out that in her younger years she had been a sculptor. I just ignored her grumpy and hateful ways, and before long I had her working again in art. It helped her change, and people were getting along with her a lot better. Other people just saw her as this hateful woman nobody could get along with, but I knew there was a reason why she was acting that way. I don't know if I would have been able to see that if I didn't have my own problems.

Lenn, who was incapacitated for years following a car accident, describes her feelings of compassion for everyone, not just those who are obviously suffering:

> It's just really deepened me as a person, increased my appreciation, and increased my compassion for people, not just people who visibly seem to be in a bad way. In truth, we're all in a bad way—one way or another. Everybody's got their own little pains, whether they're emotional, physical, whatever, and we're just all out here being human beings . . . and it's hard being a human being. So it just increases my awareness and my sensitivity to that. Before, if I

got impatient about something, if somebody wasn't moving fast enough, I'd say, "Why isn't this person moving faster?" Now I'm thinking, *Well, they might be sick, they might not be feeling well,* any number of things. I just have a greater awareness that people are operating with challenges, and I'm not so quick to judge and get angry about things if they're just not going as fast as I want them to.

Patti has lived with the pain of multiple myeloma for many years. She describes what wisdom means to her and her experience in tutoring a student:

I think wisdom means having a genuine, compassionate under-standing of what's going on around me. You know, looking at other people's struggles and being able to really feel their struggle. Today I was tutoring some gal—she was Chinese. I could feel her struggling with the kinds of things that are so common to Asian speakers who are learning English. Instead of getting impatient with her, I could just feel her struggle and was able to make her see what she needed to do without her feeling put down. I guess that's a more compas-sionate look of life, and I would never have had it if this pain hadn't hit me over the head and made me slow down. I would have gone on being the jerk I always was. Ugh, I was terrible. I'm really glad I had this second chance.

The wisdom narratives show that living through suffering can bring more gratitude, greater empathy, and deepened compassion for others. The healing process often involves consciously setting a positive course and taking many positive steps. In the next chapter, we look at the inner work of self-reflection, prayer, and meditation.

11. Quiet Reflection, Meditation, and Mindfulness

Look within. Within is the fountain of the good, and it will ever bubble up, if thou wilt ever dig. —MARCUS AURELIUS

Adopt the pace of nature; her secret is patience. —RALPH WALDO EMERSON

THE CONTEMPLATIVE PRACTICES of quiet reflection, meditation, and prayer have been practiced for millennia in many of the world's spiritual traditions. Today these techniques are taught for health benefits. They are sometimes called self-regulation, progressive relaxation, or mindfulness-based stress reduction (MBSR). The stories of people working through adversity provide many examples of quiet reflection, meditation, and mindfulness. Some of our participants found peace through prayer and meditation, some by working in a garden, and some simply found moments of stillness in the course of daily life. In this chapter we look at the ways these practices quietly supported people in relieving suffering, finding answers to profound existential questions, and moving toward wholeness—from personal, spiritual, and scientific perspectives.

Studies show that cultivating peace and tranquility has important health benefits. Deep relaxation calms the stress circuits of the brain, which become overactivated during extended periods of distress (Benson 1979). Too much stress affects our capacity to pay attention fully and to do our best in challenging circumstances. This was scientifically established over a century ago (Diamond 2005), but you probably do not need scientific evidence to believe this. We have all experienced the

difficulty of being in situations that require our full attention when we
are overly stressed.

The Relaxation Response

Herbert Benson, a Harvard cardiologist, for decades has studied the
effects of relaxation, prayer, and meditation on health and well-being.
In a talk he gave to a group of cardiologists, he joked about how, in
earlier times, he would sneak meditators into his laboratory after dark,
afraid of what his colleagues might think if he conducted these studies
during the day. This attitude has changed in recent years. Many labora-
tories now study the neurophysiology of meditation, with newsworthy
results and increased funding from the National Institutes of Health
(Lutz, Greischar, et al. 2004). Benson summarizes his findings on the
physiological effects and health benefits of prayer and meditation:

> For more than 25 years laboratories at the Harvard Medi-
> cal School have systematically studied the benefits of mind/
> body interactions. The research established that when a per-
> son engages in a repetitive prayer, word, sound or phrase and
> when intrusive thoughts are passively disregarded, a specific
> set of physiologic changes ensue. There is decreased metabo-
> lism, heart rate, rate of breathing and distinctive slower brain
> waves. These changes are the opposite of those induced by
> stress and are an effective therapy in a number of diseases that
> include hypertension, cardiac rhythm irregularities, many
> forms of chronic pain, insomnia, infertility, the symptoms
> of cancer and AIDS, premenstrual syndrome, anxiety and
> mild and moderate depression. In fact, to the extent that any
> disease is caused or made worse by stress, to that extent this
> physiological state is an effective therapy. (Benson 1997, 1695)

Benson's studies point to the universality of these experiences,
whether it be prayer, chanting, or repeating a mantra. There are some

differences in techniques that may be helpful in understanding the relationship of meditation and mindfulness. Later in the chapter we examine these differences. For now, let's look at the similarities in prayer and meditative practices across the world's spiritual traditions.

PRAYER AND MEDITATION IN THE SPIRITUAL TRADITIONS

In 2000 a conversation took place in New York City among five spiritual leaders from the Christian, Hindu, Muslim, Jewish, and Buddhist traditions at the Cathedral of St. John the Divine (*Five Masters of Meditation* 2002). They discussed the nature of prayer and meditation, looking for the commonalities among their practices. This all-day event gave the attendees an opportunity to participate in many different kinds of prayer and meditation, and perhaps forge a common bond. Feelings of oneness and connectedness were described in the Christian practice of Communion and compared to Muslim practices during the month of Ramadan and the Jewish word *shalom*, which means "completeness" or "wholeness" (in addition to "peace"). The Muslim leader observed that the unity and facial expressions of Christians returning from Communion seemed to him just like the faces of a group of Muslims kneeling together during Ramadan. He also remarked that he spent a good part of his life discussing and debating the differences among the world's religions. Now in his older years he has come to realize that the languages may differ, but the practices all have the same goal: the experience of oneness, unity, and wholeness.

The Jewish leader described meditation as "a very good, deep scrub." It "cleans the mind and opens the heart." From the Hindu perspective, "the mind is a mirror." When the mind is "calm and clear," you can see yourself. No agitation. "Keep the mind calm. Keep the mind clear." The Buddhist leader focused on "being in the present" and finding your "true home."

Many different kinds of meditation were practiced throughout the day. For example, the Hindu leader offered the meditation of focusing

on a rose and gave humorous examples of the mind attempting to stay
focused on the rose.

> After a moment's contemplation, what happens to the mind? It
> starts to think. "That guy gave me the rose." [A brief silence.] "I
> haven't seen him since then." [Another brief silence.] "I wonder if I
> should call him?" [Laughter.] "What happened to the rose? Go back
> to the rose."

All the leaders gave instruction on what to do *when*, not *if*, the mind
wanders. Gently bring your attention back to the breath, the mantra, or
the rose. Also, to help calm the mind, first calm and balance the body.

The Jewish leader led the group in a singing meditation with the
group rhythmically moving their bodies and snapping their fingers.
Chanting certain words or mantra syllables is common practice in
many traditions. Involving the body in calming, soothing movements
helps the mind come to rest. The Buddhist monk led a walking meditation around the cathedral, each person slowly and silently walking in
rhythmic unity.

Sue, who had a damaged nerve in her elbow, began a meditation
practice to help with her pain and found immediate relief:

> I started doing meditation and found that during just the breathing,
> the very simple breathing exercise, almost immediately it was just
> amazing how much better it felt. It was just like this window of relief.
> Plus I was just intrigued that I could make my body do this thing: I
> could just breathe and I would feel warm and I would feel okay, and
> *Wow, what else could I do?*

The sense of being intrigued by her injury and her joy in learning
was palpable. She became fascinated with what was happening in her
painful arm and rapidly learned to engage in short periods of meditation to calm her pain and gain a bit of strength to help her keep going.

Some participants in our study said that sitting in meditation is just

too frustrating. Some found it easier to focus their attention on movement, like walking, breathing, making art, or taking care of a garden.

The Frustrations of Sitting Quietly

Helen is a pain patient with a very stressful life and a long history of
back pain. She decided to stop having injections and unsuccessful surgeries and tried meditation in hopes of finding some relief.

> I can't concentrate like that. My mind wanders too much. I try and
> try and can't. I cannot do sitting meditation; it drives me crazy. But
> walking meditation works for me, and eating meditation works for
> me—mindfulness in general.
>
> It's very difficult for me to do. I tried to do it. I have tapes. I have
> everything, but one minute you're there, the next minute you're
> just sort of dancing around, your mind cannot be calm. I've gone
> to all sorts of people. One therapist was so excited, she would say,
> "Let's just do it for five minutes. Just let me talk to you. Let's be
> comfortable." Everything was perfect. I finally felt that I was getting
> into it. Then she said, "Get rid of all those crazy monkeys in your
> tree." And instantly all I could see was monkeys dancing around in
> a tree. I thought, *Well, that didn't work.* So I do try deep breathing,
> that's very helpful.

Meditation in Art and in the Garden

Monica developed arthritis as a young adult and finds getting involved
in art to be an effective pain reliever. Many other pain participants also
cultivated focused attention in artistic endeavors and gained relief from
pain in these meditative activities. Monica reported,

> I started to do these little mandalas, just something I could do in
> maybe ten or fifteen minutes. When I'm playing with color, it's as
> if my mind is fully absorbed in that activity and I can transcend

other things. Through art, I can go to another place. It's like a visual meditation.

In chapter 10, Jenny recounted the gratitude she feels for being able to return to farming after years of recovering from a back injury. She finds moments of deep concentration and stillness working in her garden.

It feels like I'm part of the creative process to grow good food and shepherd it along. That level of observation is like meditation. There is nothing else that I can be thinking about and doing and paying attention to—a plant's growth and hoeing the weeds in between the two plants that are four inches apart and needing to navigate my hoe quickly and thoroughly and not kill the plant that is supposed to be growing there. Nothing else can come into my head: I have to focus on that. For me it is a meditative process and it just gets me in tune with being.

Self-Reflection

Personal reflection is another way to describe rumination, the term that Calhoun and Tedeschi use in their theory of posttraumatic growth. Reflection is a time-consuming process, since calmly turning our attention to a difficult circumstance may not yield answers right away. A steady habit of the mind eventually produces a resolution. Common to all the practices is the initial quieting of the mind to calm the stress, and then devoting some quiet attention to the problem. Over time, this process can bring insight, resolution, and peace.

Maurice realized that uncontrolled stress from his back injury made his pain worse, and he was determined to live well with pain. He exercises regularly and keeps his stress and pain in check, tuning in to himself and listening to what his body is saying. Maurice is a great example of choosing a positive course and holding oneself to that course. His times of personal reflection often lead to an insight that comes to him, maybe even days afterward.

> For me a lot of it is just personal reflection—spending some time with myself, just asking myself, *Is that the right thing to have said? Did I do the right thing, or is there a way I could have done it better?* I might be walking somewhere someday, and suddenly I see something, and it relates to what I was thinking about. *Oh, that's the answer.*

Dr. S describes the difficulties of communication and decision making in end-of-life care. In her case, another doctor thought she failed to give a treatment that may have extended the life of an elderly man. She describes praying as "giving it over" and recalls her mother's advice to let God help solve the problem:

> In times of doubt and struggle, my mother would say, "You pray the rosary and you give it to God and then he helps to figure it out," which is probably partly true but at least that mantra of praying and giving it over gives you some peace of mind. So it certainly does help.

Earlier we related the story of Dr. C, who had the courage to ask her patient for forgiveness after contributing to a delay in the diagnosis of his cancer. Eventually she experienced greater appreciation, empathy, and the softening of her heart with kindness. Here she explains the process of learning to forgive herself; months of self-reflection and talking with others came to fruition in a moment of prayer:

> It took effort and work. I went to my pastor, I went to talk some more with my colleagues. It was an ongoing process. I reflected, and that took a while. It took time. It was like water on a rock. It was a definite moment. I remember the day I talked with my patient and the day in the hospital room—that's very vividly clear to me.

Then something happened during a prayer. I felt a sensation and a calming—it was a definite event. I felt a sense of peace. I didn't hear a voice or anything, but I just had this inner knowledge: "Be still and know I am God and I give you my grace."

Like a rock, a problem can seem solid and permanent—impervious to something as light as a prayer. But over time, just like the steady movement of water on a rock, prayer can transform a situation that seems hard and unyielding and bring about peaceful understanding and grace.

Dr. C goes on to talk about the importance of staying clear and attentive. Recognizing her limitations goes hand in hand with taking responsibility for being conscious and mindful.

We have people's precious lives in our hands. We cannot be distracted because our kid is sick or our car is broken. All those problems of daily living have to be left behind when we walk through that office door. We have to be laser-focused, and that's really hard to do, every day, all day, because we are human. We do think about if our kid is sick, or if we're having problems. We do get distracted and may not be so alert to some sign or something as we should be. So we have to be conscious and mindful that we have to be on. We have to turn that switch on when we walk in there—when we're talking to people and we hold their lives in our hands. We can't be lackadaisical or lazy. We have to be sharp.

THE NEUROSCIENCE OF QUIET REFLECTION, MEDITATION, AND MINDFULNESS

Recent developments in neuroscience give us a window on what is happening in the brain during moments of quiet reflection and meditation and help us understand how these states restore what might be considered our most valuable renewable resource: clear and focused attention.

Having the ability to clear the mind of stressful thoughts and emotions is usually the beginning of any meditation practice. This can be very challenging at times. Teachers often tell students that clearing the mind for even half a cycle of breath can be taken as an achievement. A little bit of success can be the start of a discipline that improves with practice.

The anterior cingulate cortex is a brain region involved in calming the emotional centers of the brain through deliberate intention. It is a hub of connectivity that serves an integrative function, coordinating our intentions, our emotional reactions, and our actions. Studies have found this circuit to be more active during meditation by experienced practitioners (Treadway, Lazar, and Didonna 2009). The practice of exerting conscious control over our emotions involves the integration of head and heart, leading to reduced suffering, an increased sense of personal strength, and feelings of loving-kindness and compassion (Hanson and Mendius 2009). The descriptions of unity, oneness, and wholeness given by the spiritual leaders can be understood as a more coordinated network of brain function, integrating parts of ourselves formerly in conflict. When we are able to calm our emotional distress through prayer, meditation, or any activity that centers us, we can then experience the peace and tranquility that are at the core of these practices.

A Network of Stillness

A recently discovered network in the brain—called the default mode network (DMN)—can give us insight into the nature of mental stillness. The DMN comprises large areas of the brain, including the medial frontal precortex and the medial parietal cortex, inside the right hemisphere, and the medial prefrontal cortex, the lateral temporal, and the lateral parietal cortex on the outside of the left hemisphere (Raichle 2010). These brain regions are relatively large and widely separated from each other. Yet during periods of inactivity, these brain regions behave in a coordinated way as if they were physically connected. It is as if members of a family living in various regions of the country were taking part in a quiet conference call.

Scientists typically study brain activity when people are actively engaged in a task, but the DMN is most active during times of rest and apparent inactivity. When we experience periods of mental stillness, this network of brain regions goes to work. The activity is very slow, with most of its energy at 0.1 cycles per second. Imagine someone beating a drum every ten seconds. During meditation the DMN is even more active than during periods of mental quiescence (Travis et al. 2010).

You have likely experienced periods of mental stillness in the course of daily life, even if you do not pray or meditate. For example, Tricia, who has been in a wheelchair since a car accident in her youth, finds that taking a long, relaxing bath is a chance to clear her mind and take a healthful break. While bathing, she loses track of time, which often happens when the mind is still and calm.

> I like trying to take some time, such as when I take a bath. I tend to be more comfortable, and if the water's nice and warm it just puts me in a more relaxed place, and that's where I'll try that. In the afternoons, I usually take a long bath—thirty minutes—and I find that even if I just close my eyes and I'm not even paying attention to how long, I'll see that I've just taken a twenty-minute break from everything. I think it's very healthy for me. I don't focus on anything. I try not to have thoughts. That works for me.

Betsy, a nurse introduced earlier, took years to recover from a car accident. She expressed deep appreciation for her recovery and compassion for the pain of others who are still in the process of healing. Here she describes the rejuvenation she feels from a moment of deep stillness:

> I remember being there and it wasn't even at church. It was just kind of quiet. Sort of just feeling like the Earth had stopped rotating. And that's the first time that I've ever felt that. And I thought, *Hmm, all is at peace.* I can get myself back to that state again if I need to. I find that stillness even in the midst of busyness. I find it

sometimes when I'm traveling, taking care of a patient, or if I'm out someplace where it's beautiful. I'm not talking about the Caribbean, just a market or something where you see artwork or those kinds of things. I've felt as if the Earth has stopped rotating; that's pretty good. I don't always need to be there, but I feel as if I could do that again if I have to. I think, in the long run, if you can take a big drink and fill your cup during those short times, then you're good to go for longer, because I wouldn't want to just always be sitting and feeling like the Earth has stopped rotating. I guess it's like a pit stop, where you stop and go again.

When Betsy recalls the rejuvenation she finds in these silent moments, she is talking about a universal human experience at the heart of the contemplative traditions. Many spiritual teachers believe that cultivating awareness of this silence makes us feel wholly present and expands our awareness of being in the moment. The noisy chatter of mental life, thinking about the past and planning the future, is stilled. This silent world within each of us has been called a vast inner space that is intensely alive and the source of pure creative intelligence. However it is described, there is agreement that the cultivation of inner stillness restores us—physically, emotionally, mentally, and spiritually. Bringing the power of stillness into our daily lives is the heart of mindfulness.

MINDFULNESS

Mindfulness depends on the ability to calm the mind, maintain focused attention, and adopt a nonjudgmental, accepting attitude. It is easy to understand how a calm, focused mind can more readily accept traumatic life experiences. But staying calm in the throes of a traumatic event is a classic case of "easier said than done." That is why the practice of mindfulness is a lifetime endeavor developed over years of practice. Jon Kabat-Zinn developed an eight-week program of mindfulness-based stress reduction (MBSR) in the context of a clinic for patients with many clinical conditions that worsen with uncontrolled stress. He encourages people listening to his guided meditations to "befriend" their pain, "putting out the welcome mat for unwanted sensations, even very intense ones" and "seeing what happens as you invite them into your field of awareness" (Kabat-Zinn 2010, CD no. 2, track no. 3).

In the study of meditation a distinction is made between open monitoring (OM) and focused attention (FA) (Raffone and Srinivasan 2010). Examples of focused attention are the meditation on the rose offered by the Hindu leader, Jenny in her garden, or the artist's absorption in colored mandalas. Studies of Buddhist monks, trained in highly focused attention, exhibited brain rhythms that became progressively more synchronized and coherent (Lutz et al. 2004). They were measured to have high-amplitude gamma waves, which can be compared to a high-intensity laser of focused attention.

Mindfulness practice is an example of open monitoring—calm and open awareness of whatever comes into attention. The practice of mindfulness is an effective way to keep stress at a healthy level and our mental function in a state of relaxed alertness. While different brain circuitry may be involved in FA and OM techniques, a natural compatibility exists between them. It has been posited that becoming proficient in focused attention supports the development of open monitoring and mindfulness. Open monitoring is thought to help in restructuring our autobiographical narrative, becoming more aware of what triggers our distress, mindfully accepting it, and thus supporting the integration into a new narrative (Lutz et al. 2008).

We introduced the concept of mindfulness in chapter 4 because the essence of mindfulness is acceptance. Developing this capacity can take time. Mindfulness instructors tell their students in the beginning stages that they don't have to enjoy the meditation practices—they just have to do them. After eight weeks the students can say if they are of any real use (Kabat-Zinn 2010). Our clinical studies and a growing base of mindfulness research support the utility of mindfulness for the management of chronic pain (Plews-Ogan et al. 2005) and many other stressful conditions (Baer 2003). Mindfulness may be best understood by practicing it, but scientific definitions are available. Mindfulness is defined as "self-regulation of attention and adopting a particular orientation toward one's experience in the present moment, an orientation that is characterized by curiosity, openness, and acceptance" (Bishop et al. 2004, 232) and "the awareness that emerges through paying attention on purpose, in the present moment, and non-judgmentally to the unfolding of experience moment by moment" (Kabat-Zinn 2003, 145). As Kabat-Zinn points out, the practice of mindfulness is historically associated with Buddhism. In Asian languages, the words for *heart* and *mind* are the same. So mindfulness translates as "an affectionate, compassionate quality within the attending, a sense of openhearted, friendly presence and interest" (145). Just as the five world spiritual leaders found commonality across contemplative traditions, mindfulness is a universal human capacity: paying attention with an open heart.

Tracey DeGregory says in the film *Choosing Wisdom*: "There is a part of you that is a witness, an observer." The observer consciousness is aware of what is happening but remains detached from the pain and suffering it is witnessing. A simple exercise in mindfulness asks you to look at your suffering. Is the part of you that is looking at your suffering itself suffering? If you can catch a glimpse, even feel a whisper of the part of you that can observe the worst pain and suffering imaginable, but that part of you is calm and simply aware of it, that is mindfulness.

Lenn, first introduced in chapter 4, has been practicing meditation for thirty years. She readily applied her meditation experience to help her heal the pain from a car accident. She notes that accepting her pain lessens her suffering, while saying no to the pain just increases its severity. Like other participants who can successfully control their pain with meditation, Lenn describes her experience with enthusiasm and a fascination for the dynamics of her inner world. She points out that she directs her calm and focused attention to the pain, "getting in there" and then feeling the waves of her painful sensation subsiding. Lenn also describes the benefits of maintaining mindful attention to become aware of the sources of stress in her life:

Another reason why meditation is great is that you can observe yourself and observe what you're doing and observe what you're thinking and your attitudes. As an example, whenever I talk to a certain person, I start getting into this kind of thing that doesn't seem so productive. Then you can move to a more positive, more productive place once you've noticed that. To me, that is what meditation does. It helps you notice those things. Because otherwise you're stuck. You'll just keep going in this loop, this endless loop. With mindfulness, you can say, "Well, I did have that experience, but maybe it could be different."

The practice of mindfulness can be described as bringing the still space of meditation into daily life. This is the space where we can quietly observe what is happening from an objective point of view. Mindfully observing our reactions gives us a greater capacity to make choices and possibly calm a stress reaction that could otherwise escalate.

Patti, who lives with the pain of bone cancer, explains how she transforms a potentially stressful experience of being stuck in traffic to an opportunity to practice mindfulness.

I learned through my practice of yoga—the discipline of learning to breathe my way through life—to take stressful things, things that would be stressors, and try to change my response to them. If I get stuck in traffic, I can use that as an opportunity to breathe and relax. Then being stuck in traffic is actually an opportunity to relax for a little bit instead of it being a stressful situation.

Patti is responding mindfully, not automatically reacting to a situation that typically causes people to feel irritation or even rage. These conscious responses are like choosing to get on one train and not another. You see the stress train arriving and the door opening, and you simply decide to let that one go down the track and choose one that will do no harm or even be beneficial. Having the awareness and control to make this choice is at the heart of mindful living. Incorporating mindfulness into daily life is choosing wisdom, which can be done in small ways every day.

Lenn and Patti have practiced meditation for many years, and the fruits of their mature practice are obvious. They both accept their pain and are aware that stress increases their level of suffering. Through mindfulness, they stay in touch with stressful reactions and change either their situations or their reactions to them. Lenn and Patti both feel compassion for the suffering of others (see chapter 10), paying attention with an open heart to their own pain and to the pain of others. That is the essence of mindfulness.

Spiritual Traditions, Neuroscience, and the Path to Wisdom

From antiquity to the present, the contemplative traditions have nourished the development of wisdom and the release from suffering. Studies of the physiological processes during these practices give us a new understanding of these ancient traditions. Together, the spiritual and scientific perspectives help illuminate the path to wisdom. During quiet reflection and meditation we develop the capacity to calm distress, which can be a significant aid in accepting difficult circumstances and reducing inner conflict. During meditation, brain rhythms become more synchronized, and channels of communication within the brain are developed. This increased integration of physiological activity is accompanied by feelings of oneness and wholeness. Reducing inner conflict and increasing integration can bring greater emotional equanimity and an expanded awareness. Now we can respond, rather than react, to life challenges. We have the capacity to create new life narratives as we welcome and reframe the stressful parts of our lives. The release from suffering comes in the awareness that we can mindfully choose to accept our life experience. It is our resistance that creates suffering. Stories of self-reflection, meditation, and mindfulness express the power of this quiet work to support our journey at every step.

12. Doing Something

Whatever you can do, or believe you can do, begin it. For boldness has genius, power, and magic in it.
—JOHANN WOLFGANG VON GOETHE

NEUROSCIENTIST ADELE DIAMOND once talked about teaching children and how we can best encourage them to learn and try new behaviors, even if they resist. "You say, 'Just do it. Just do it fully and do it and you'll get something out of the doing. The act, the doing, is absolutely critical and will transform you'" (Diamond 2009). This notion of doing something fully, no matter how much we would prefer to stay under the covers or take the easy road, is an important step in healing. We saw this in the examples of "stepping in" in chapter 5, where patients and physicians took a first step toward positive change and wisdom. Making positive changes and helping others were important facilitators of growth for patients and physicians. For some of the latter, their experience precipitated a whole new career focus on patient safety. For others, teaching medical students and residents how to avoid mistakes or practice safely was important to their healing.

For the pain patients, taking charge of their own recovery and wellness was crucial. For many, it was healing to help others who were suffering with pain. Helping others who were enduring some hardship helped to put their own suffering in perspective, making it more tolerable. Helping others also gave their own situation meaning.

Making Positive Changes

Figure Out What Happened

When an error occurs, an important and natural step for physicians is to find out why the error happened and then take steps to ensure that it never happens again. When an insulin dosing error caused by poor handwriting resulted in a terrible outcome for a patient, one physician made immediate changes to his practice.

> Number one, I never use the letter *U* as an abbreviation for insulin anymore. Second, I always insist that two people review my dosing. Once the nurse draws up insulin, you have to have another nurse or a physician check and make sure that you agree that this was the dose that was written. We needed to change the system. To my knowledge this has never happened since.

After a wrong-site surgery, a surgeon knew he had to figure out why the mistake had occurred.

> When I got over the shock of what had happened and was sitting at my desk at the end of that day, my thoughts were, *Okay, figure out what happened.* I went through the process that I normally go through to avoid wrong-site surgeries, and I decided, *Okay, there's some things I need to do.* At that point, in addition to marking the "Yes" on the correct part, I changed my marking strategy so that when we're doing multiple sites, I'm going to have a mark or an arrow or something to point me to the correct ones. And I added a step to write "No" on the spots where I would do the wrong one. This is all in magic marker. It's probably kept me from doing the wrong site God knows how many times. And I have the patient put the mark on her own body part the night before. No one knows better than the patient where her surgery is.

Once a doctor figures out why and how the medical error occurred, the logical next step is to share that knowledge with others, even if it means publicly acknowledging the mistake. Dr. B was devastated when one of his first patients during his internship died. No one on the team could come up with a diagnosis, and, because of that, the patient did not receive surgery in time. An autopsy revealed a bowel ischemia.

> One of the things that I have done since then is that I've told the story. Not the emotional part of the story—partially that—but I've told the clinical story probably fifty times. I'd use it as a teaching case so that this might not happen to someone else. At my third-year residents' conference, I did a sort of literature review on this and did a write-up, and then I used that handout to teach students and residents for twenty years. But you can see why I might want to do my project on it, why I consider myself a minor expert on the condition. That was part of my coping skills: to learn about it and say, "How can I help other people?"

Another physician, Dr. U, introduced in chapter 8, shifted her practice after a wrong diagnosis to include more teaching of young doctors, partly as a way to share her experience. Her error involved "framing" a patient incorrectly, something that happens often in medicine.

> I framed this guy as a young guy with the flu, rather than a drug addict with a fever. So I know precisely where I went wrong. I didn't have a knowledge deficit; I fell into one of these traps. And I think when you teach people, nothing beats a good example.

One doctor chose a rather dramatic moment to share with colleagues, resident physicians, and students his story of a missed diagnosis:

> I used this example when I got an award for clinical work. I used this story as part of my acceptance speech. The point was we're never as great as we think we are or as bad as we think we are. We're human. That was the first time I'd told that story to an audience, so that was the first time I'd really exposed it.

Some physicians even go so far as to try to address the institutional
and wider issues that have a direct or indirect impact on their experience. In the film, Dr. Jo Shapiro saw that there was no forum for
peers to help one another through the aftermath of a bad outcome, so
she established a peer support program for health care providers. That
program has become a model nationwide. Several physicians became
involved in patient safety programs in their hospital or practice as a
result. According to Dr. Shapiro:

> I see the importance of improving quality of care. To me the solu-
> tion to both of these problems was to have the appropriate systems
> in place. Systems are like the ropes that a rock climber uses. If you
> have appropriate systems in place, it gives you more freedom. Some
> people worry that if you make everything so systematized, it doesn't
> give you the freedom to make the choices you need to make. In my
> mind, if I have the systems in place, then I don't have to have all the
> details in place. It gives you more processing room in your brain; to
> use a computer analogy, it frees up more RAM. So I think quality is
> important. And I think it's important for everybody to be involved.

Dr. T, the surgeon whose case ended in a difficult lawsuit, became
involved in reforming malpractice policy in the United States. She even
served on a roundtable with then-president George W. Bush.

> There's got to be reform in medical liability or the cost will keep
> going up. I think slowly but surely it'll change. It started as a coping
> strategy, but it turned into kind of a mission.

Strategizing Recovery

Just as the physicians needed to develop an error prevention strategy,
many patients who were successful at managing or adapting to their
pain explained the importance of developing a plan or strategy for their
recovery. Patients needed strategies that would enable them to reduce or
stop their medications. One patient said, "It just seemed really impor-

tant to find a way to feel better without having to put something into my body all the time." We believe that creating a strategy might be helpful, in part, because it provides an opportunity for patients to look up and away from the pain, to envision a better future for themselves. It is also empowering to recognize that what you do matters, and remaining passive or accepting the role of victim is not the only option.

Researchers de Sales Turner and Helen Cox interviewed people who had suffered traumatic injuries—car and motorcycle accidents, and falling off a house. In their study of recovery, they reported findings similar to ours:

> The importance of strategizing recovery cannot be empha-
> sized enough, as the findings of this study clearly demon-
> strate. The participants strongly vocalized their need to be
> involved in devising their own recovery pathway, identifying
> that not being involved made them feel as if they were not
> important to those who were delivering care. (2004, 34)

Kathy, who suffered from migraines, told us many things about successful strategizing, including, "Be proactive. Ask for what you need. Get a routine." She pointed out that you "really have to work at it. It's taking the opportunity when you see it."

When asked about turning points in her own recovery, Sue Holden, who appears in the film, said,

> A couple things, maybe three things. One, finding a doctor who
> believed that my pain was real and there was a way to deal with it
> and who didn't keep telling me, "Just keep taking Tylenol—you'll
> be better." Two, the meditation, because that really gave me a lot of
> personal control; if I couldn't make the pain go away, I could get it
> to a point where I could handle it. And, *Wow, what else could I do?*
> Those were probably the two biggest things. Then, feeling that I had
> a strategy to deal with it—a strategy, like I had some things I could
> use. I had a doctor who believed me and who was working with me

to try to figure out how we can handle this. So I began to see that it would be resolved. It would take time, but it would be resolved.

Sue also shared the feeling of empowerment that came from taking some degree of control over her own recovery and healing, through learning to get relief from her pain with breath work and meditation:

Meanwhile, I started doing meditation. Actually I took a beginning class and found that during the breathing, the very simple breathing exercise, a hand that had been really cold and in severe pain felt better. As soon as I started doing the breathing exercises, it came pretty naturally. It was just amazing how much better it felt almost immediately. It was like this window of relief. It felt very empowering, because I could then do something about it. I had control, and I found that it worked for other things, too. Since then, I coached my mom.

Trying Something New

We talked to individuals who shared a wealth of experience about adopting new strategies for self-care and healing. Betty suffered a broken elbow and severe whiplash in a car accident. The pain in her neck was like someone "sticking a knife in me." People told her she looked like a turkey, she had become so distorted. Her mood was miserable, too, because of the pain and having to give up the things she enjoyed so much, like quilting, biking, and hiking in the mountains. She couldn't sleep, and the pain was controlling her life. She remembers going for a walk with her husband, and he said, "See that bird up there?" She became angry that he'd forgotten she couldn't lift her head. Betty explains,

I wasn't being the creative or active person that I was, and I wasn't happy. I would cry at the drop of a hat; I was snapping people's heads off. I mean, I was going back and apologizing to people at work. I was apologizing to my husband.

She tried medications. She tried physical therapy and a chiropractor, but nothing helped. At one point she considered surgery, but the surgeon told her there was nothing he could do for her pain. One day, she asked her doctor, "What do you think about yoga?" Betty didn't know the first thing about yoga, but her doctor said he loved yoga for his patients, and now she sees that her turning point was the day she said, "I'm going to reach out to something that I'm unsure of."

> The yoga, I didn't know enough about it. I thought it was "out there." My husband said, "Oh my God, what is she doing?" But I thought it was worth trying. I went into it with an open mind, and I remember walking into the class the first time and not knowing what the heck we're gonna do. I met with the instructor when I signed the release, and she said, "Let pain be your guide." There were some positions that I couldn't go into, that weren't comfortable. Then in time, she said, "Look at you. You're able to do that. You're holding it longer!"

The lesson of letting pain be her guide helped Betty get back to the other activities she loves, whether it's raking leaves or riding her bike. Her doctor finally told her, "You can resume all those things you enjoy, but let pain be your guide. If it hurts, don't do as much." She told him she loved to ride her bike, but the compression in the handlebars gave her pain in her shoulders.

> The doctor asked, "How far are you riding?" I said, "I used to do seventy-five to one hundred miles a day." He said, "Whoa, try eight or ten miles. If it's screaming at five, that's enough for that day." I was learning moderation, learning acceptance that maybe I can't do the distance I did, but accepting what I can do. I really feel it was accepting it—the yoga with the relaxation—and helping me sort of get into balance. And building my core strength, and realizing how counter-stretching had played a role in helping to release that tension that I had all the time.

Betty continues to do well and attributes her willingness to "try something that I didn't even know anything about" to what changed the way she deals with her pain.

Betty turned to yoga, but others turned to many other strategies, including journaling or creative writing. Sue began writing as a way to document her pain, and although it also served a healing purpose, the documentation itself was useful when she met with her physicians.

> The writing really did help. But when I started, I thought I was just going to document. Then I would start writing about my feelings and the darkness. I would finally get up off the bed, and I would make myself write something about that day because I guess it was therapeutic. It was also a way for me to look back as time went on, and I was really glad I had done it: to look back and say, "This really did happen to me—it really was this bad." I wasn't crazy in my head for thinking I was in this much pain.

Others developed an appreciation for art and music. Mary, one of the study's fibromyalgia patients, explained a turning point for her. "I discovered poetry, and I discovered that art helped me, and I discovered that theater helped me. I love literature, I love music, so all these things helped me, too." All these healing strategies included some combination of self-care activities that worked for the patient, such as exercise, sleep and rest, yoga, meditation, and water therapies, such as soaking in mineral hot springs (or Epsom-salt baths), Jacuzzi therapy, and exercising in warm-water pools.

Nature was a powerful healing force, including gardening and simply walking in nature. Patricia, whose fibromyalgia pain was so severe she couldn't sleep or hold a book, finally found relief in nature.

> Wherever I live, I always have to have—aside from indoors where I meditate—a place outdoors where it's energy-refreshing. A couple blocks from my house there is a view overlooking the bay, and I

take my dog and walk over there and just sit and feel the breeze and watch boats, feel the sunlight on me, and pet my dog. My dog is part of my recovery. She is so sweet and loving. I feel revitalized just being outdoors and in the sunlight.

There was also a lot of talk among patients about how important it was to keep moving—physically and metaphorically. Sue Holden found an interesting way to do this:

That first year, my next-door neighbor, who was thirteen at the time, would come over. I lived on a one-acre, mostly wooded lot, and she and I would walk around my yard every single day. I would point to rocks and she would dig them up, and I built stone walls. I mean, little rocks, big rocks, every rock I could find in that yard. And it was fun, because she and I did it together. Something else was also at the root of it. I couldn't drive anywhere, and I wasn't going to sit in the house and think about how bad I felt. Instead, I thought, *I'm going to build something.*

It was fun. I was outside, I wasn't able to do major hikes or anything like that. But I could walk around that yard with her and she'd pick up the rocks with me. It was frustrating when we realized there were no more rocks left. We could have kept going.

Helping Others

In their research, Elizabeth Salick and Carl Auerbach found that helping others was a key factor in healing. "Growth also followed from being involved in giving something back, which came from feeling empowered to contribute to a social or world community. Half the sample reported a desire to contribute or give back to their community in some way" (2000, 1032). It was often because the people had experienced illness or medical error, and the experience allowed them to share with others the wisdom they had gained. In many cases, the patients turned around and helped people who had similar conditions or experiences, and some simply helped others in need. Seeing the difficulties that other people face provided a wider perspective.

Sue Holden, for example, was able to teach her mother how to cope with pain:

> She had had a fractured shoulder and hip and was in enormous pain. I was able to show her the breathing techniques and to tell her from my experience how they had helped me. She was willing to try it, and it did help a little bit. It was a way I could also bond with her and try to be a support to her, which was very gratifying for me as well.

As she has healed, Sue also has helped others, including the children she met overseas who live in a garbage dump, and she has gained an appreciation for her own circumstances.

> I think I have a deeper appreciation for the fact that at least I have an option to heal and get well. Some of these kids have nothing.

Helping others was a common theme among patients as well as physicians. Patients told us of their volunteer work, advocacy activities, and willingness to serve as role models for others struggling with illness or injury. Not only does the work provide distraction from the pain, as Sue found, it also helps to put one's own suffering in perspective.

Emily says that coping with her pain has been part of her "personal redemption," and that she is now attuned to the feelings and needs of others in a way she had never been. "Had I not had this issue with the pain in my life, I might not have identified with the pain of other people," she says. Although she is living in a shelter and saving money to afford her own apartment, she has made it a mission to learn more about the needs of people in northern Uganda, sending what little money she can to charities that work there, and doing what she can to increase local awareness about their plight. She also turns her attention to the needs of the people in her neighborhood:

Even though I have a semi-disability, I spend some of my time doing things for other people. Sometimes that means using the educational skills I have as a network engineer—I have advanced computer skills. I help people learn how to use computers for free. Recently I helped an elderly neighbor learn to use her computer and the Internet, and she wanted to pay me. I suggested that she find a charity and give what she wanted to that charity. Of course, I had her look up charities on the Internet! It takes a lot of my attention from the pain, and it gives me satisfaction.

David was diagnosed with Parkinson's disease and neuropathy in the same year. A recovering alcoholic and drug addict, he had just completed his dream of becoming a counselor. A few months before his diagnosis he had finished his graduate work and started a job helping substance abusers in a court-ordered drug rehab program. He was devastated when his physician and his employer suggested that he consider early retirement. A man with a strong work ethic, David had missed over thirty days of work in six months due to pain and stress. He retired, but eventually he found another way to use the skills he had acquired in pursuit of his dream.

I have used my counseling skills to do outreach work in the community. I established a Parkinson's disease group. It has provided support and education to other people in the area with Parkinson's disease, their family members, and friends. Each year we have hosted a symposium. I would encourage anyone with an illness to seek out support groups, attend conferences, or do whatever it takes to meet other people who are dealing with similar medical conditions.

Barbara, a fibromyalgia patient, also underscores the value of volunteering.

Put things in your life to look forward to. Get out of yourself. Go to a community support center. You think you got problems? See the hand that those folks have been dealt, and how some of them have joy in their life. Go do something. Volunteer.

As the journey through adversity increased their capacity for compassion, patients and physicians both brought this caring and empathy to their lives and work. Physicians talked about being less judgmental toward other physicians who had made mistakes, and it also made them more compassionate and better able to connect with their patients. Dr. Jamie Redgrave, speaking in the film, talks about sharing her own diabetes diagnosis with some of her patients. One physician who had struggled with substance abuse following her error was able to share with her patients her experience with addiction and recovery:

Working with addiction patients we get great outcomes, and it's because I know where they are coming from. I understand what they are feeling. For many of them I don't have problems sharing my own experience. I don't do it with all of them, but with many I share my own experience, which lets them identify a little bit. So maybe they work a little bit harder. But most of my patients do very well.

Helping by Teaching

One way of developing meaning from a difficult experience is in sharing hard-fought knowledge with others. Patients and physicians were generous and willing to pass along not only the pragmatic lessons they had learned, but also the deeper wisdom they had gleaned along their journey. For physicians, sometimes it was as straightforward as telling the story of their mistake to young physicians so that they would never repeat the same medical error. Many patients took opportunities to share techniques and therapies that worked well for them. Mary, who has fibromyalgia, extols the virtues of distracting herself and thought others might find it helpful as well:

Try to find something that lets you not think about the pain so much. With me, for example, if I go out driving at midday, I'm going to hit traffic and I'm going to run into people, and that's going to make me angry and that's going to fuel my physical discomfort, which will exacerbate my pain. So I just shut the door. I won't go out. Find something that will help you do that. With me, it's swimming, the theater, locking myself up and reading or watching a movie. In other words, distract yourself. That's the only way I could suggest because otherwise you're constantly feeding on it and feeding off it, and it makes you feel worse. And the more you feel mentally worse, the more you're going to feel the pain—the physical pain.

Other patients offered encouragement. Some went further, teaching deeper lessons. Sue Holden says,

It took advocating for myself, doing it personally, for me to really test myself and to know that I could do it and hopefully to be able to encourage others to advocate for themselves.

As a young physician, Dr. K was shown compassion by her teacher when she made a mistake—the sutured cut that became infected. She has been very intentional about sharing that same compassion with her patients and her students. Her experience with error also had a tremendous impact on her view of the world and her place in it, and she tries to impart this to her patients, many of whom are college students.

This is all fleeting. It's helped me keep the big picture of life in mind, and it's really helped me relate to my patients in helping them keep the big picture of life in mind, rather than dealing with a small problem they have. At the end of the day, if they got a little ankle sprain, it is a problem for them, but in the big picture, it's all about perspective, right? Think about Sudan, think about Darfur, and think about all these kids dying there and think about all that you have—everything you've been blessed with. I remind them about this stuff. This experience has made me very humble, and I can relate that humility to them and give them some perspective. When my professor gave me this perspective, I was able to translate that perspective into sharing with someone else. This relatively small mistake changed the way I feel about things. It's amazing how a little incident in your life can really change things for you.

Dr. B had a very different experience. He did not receive support or compassion from his attendings or supervising physicians when his patient died. It took him many years to get beyond a feeling of betrayal and disappointment. He says, however, that it crystallized his sense of himself as a teacher. He described what kind of teacher, mentor, and doctor he did *not* want to become:

> I guess that's the unanswered question, and the answer is one I am trying to live my way into, or trying to help out with. When I am on the wards, I try to be very attentive to that. And in clinic I try to radiate some kindness and humanity toward the residents.

When asked why they wanted to participate in the Wisdom in Medicine study, physicians and patients expressed a desire to help and teach others. Talking to the interviewer, who then might use their story to help others, was another way to do something, to allow something positive to come from their adversity. When Betty saw the advertisement for research participants in her local paper, she thought,

> *There are others who need to know what I've learned. It's not a pill bottle, it's not going to the surgeon who's knife-happy. It's what can I do to change it.* My husband says, "That is you."

Sue Holden wanted to share her story of coping with chronic pain, not only in the research, but also in the film.

> I feel like I've lived with the situation positively, so it's not as forceful. It's still that background noise, but it's not as forceful. If it could help someone else, if it's training physicians or looking at how we treat

patients or looking at doctor-patient relationships, any of those things—if I can be one little voice that somehow helps in that, then that's good. It also adds to the meaning of what my own experience has been, in that it's not just me and a few of my friends and my husband knowing, but I feel like something good has come out of all of this, or is still coming out of this. It's an evolving thing.

In this chapter we've explored the various ways that just doing something—whether helping others or making positive changes—can facilitate growth after adversity. The Adele Diamond passage we began with emphasizes the importance of *doing*, whether that doing feels easy or comfortable. In the interview, Diamond shared an example about helping her son with his homework and music lessons. She told him to just do them with his whole heart, and if he did that, he would be transformed in the doing. Simply in doing, in helping, in making small changes, transformation can occur. In the next chapter, we see this same idea taken to another level as we examine the role that spirituality, forgiveness, and doing the right thing plays in people's healing and growth.

13. Spirituality, Forgiveness, and Doing the Right Thing

There are two ways to live your life. One is as though nothing is a miracle. The other is as though everything is a miracle.
—ALBERT EINSTEIN

True goodness, true responsibility, true justice, a true sense of things, all these grow from roots that go much deeper than the world of our transitory earthly schemes. This is a message that speaks to us from the very heart of human spirituality.
—VÁCLAV HAVEL

The evocation of some spiritual aspiration, some concept of God, of "Fall" and "Grace," some sense of transcendence, some sense of presence in a vast universe, arises after we are aware of our humanity. —RICHARD BELL

THE EXPERIENCE of adversity—whether physical pain, emotional pain, loss, or failure—has the universal effect of making us acutely aware of our own humanity. In that realization we come face-to-face with questions of meaning, order, justice, and our place in the world. Our spiritual and moral beliefs can be challenged by the experience of adversity, but they can also help us cope and change positively as we navigate those difficult experiences.

In chapter 10 we focused on the role of gratitude and compassion in helping people move through difficult experiences. In the following pages we explore the role that spirituality and forgiveness played in people's responses to the challenges they faced.

Spirituality

Spirituality and posttraumatic growth are connected. But as Kenneth Pargament and colleagues (2006) point out, we're not exactly clear as to what that connection means. What about spirituality can facilitate growth? Is there a kind of spirituality that presents a challenge to growth or that can stand in the way of growth in some people?

As Pargament notes, spirituality can be a double-edged sword when it comes to dealing with adversity. On the one hand, it can provide a way for us to understand and help us cope well. On the other hand, it can be a stumbling block to healing when our previously held beliefs no longer suffice. Notions of a compassionate, loving, but all-powerful God are called into question in the face of extreme and undeserved suffering. Beliefs about some cosmic order to the universe and notions of justice are severely tested by situations of untimely death or unrelenting pain.

Dr. MJ relates a situation in which she struggled with her own faith after watching one of her patients lose a daughter to a brain aneurysm:

> I guess I was sort of mad at God. I mean, I just didn't see the justice in it at all.

At the same time, though, she explains that the faith and the grace displayed by the mother was so inspiring to her:

> They were so appreciative of everything that everybody did at every point along the line. Usually with patients there's some aspect of care that they have a gripe with, even if it's the cafeteria. But these folks just didn't. They have a very strong faith and they felt that things had happened for a reason and their daughter was in a good place. I don't know. I couldn't have done it.

A pediatric surgeon reflected that his faith was challenged, and that it wasn't as comfortable as before, but it remained a source of strength.

I'm not as comfortable with my "spirituality" now as I was ten years ago. I wonder what it is all about, why it happens, etc. I don't know how to understand it. I just know that they say bad things happen to good people; I've seen a lot of very good people have the trials of Job. Do I understand that spiritually? No. But I don't know that I could cope with it unless I had some level of spirituality. That's a hard one.

Kathy, who suffered with migraines, struggled with her spirituality, finding it both disconcerting and comforting.

As far as spirituality goes, it has gone both ways. I spent some of the time wanting to know why God afflicted me with this, the rest of the time saying there must be a reason. I'm just back and forth on that one.

In the Wisdom through Adversity study, we examined the relationship between spirituality, posttraumatic growth, and wisdom through a series of questionnaires as well as in our interviews. The questionnaire results suggest a connection between spirituality, posttraumatic growth, and wisdom. Exemplars in the study scored high on spirituality in both the physician and the patient groups. The narrative interview data help us understand a bit more about what that connection might be. Not all patients or physicians, though, described themselves as spiritual, but many did, and the majority of those who did found their spirituality to be important in coping with this difficult circumstance. Spirituality had different meanings for different people. For many it was not "religious," in that it had nothing to do with organized religion or even with God. A number of patients mentioned other types of spiritual practices, such as yoga.

Lauren, who suffered with migraines for years, would not describe herself as religious, but meditation and yoga provided a spiritual dimension for her that was very helpful.

I'm not really religious in a fundamental sense, but I think I've always been spiritual. I've learned the value of relaxation. So I practice meditation and yoga, and I think that's made a huge difference.

For others, spirituality had to do with nature. Scott suffered from terrible back pain that resulted in hospitalization. He describes himself as an agnostic and has a generally negative reaction to religion. But he has a spiritual connection to nature, an appreciation of and a connection to nature that resulted from his struggle with pain.

With me, the way I use the term "spirituality" is just an awareness of everything around me and the living beings and how it all functions, how it all ties in together. I'll walk out the door and look at the lawn. I look at the bugs in it, I look at the birds on it, the things that play in it, how it grows, everything. I never did that before. I've never really looked at it, I guess, with such grandeur before. Never appreciated it.

Others approached spirituality in its broadest definition: a sense of something greater than the self. For some physicians and patients, spirituality was a humanistic notion that evoked an understanding of the other as part of a deeper human striving for meaning and an understanding of ourselves as part of a larger whole. Sue Holden says,

I've always felt that there's this connectedness, which I call "spirituality." There's this *something* that's definitely a whole lot bigger than just me. I believe in grace. And I believe it's amazing and very empowering. So, yes, it's played a role in the sense that I think it does help you through the rough spots. It does help you appreciate where you are—this one little face in the sea of faces that are all of mankind over all of time. You're one little experience—valid, but still one, connected somehow. You're part of a whole. There's something out there that somehow binds us. It's a way of reflecting, a way of understanding where you fit into it, a way of drawing some strength just because there is such a thing as grace that helps you as you go through the hard times and hopefully also helps you appreciate the good times, helps you handle things in a way that you can be kind to others.

So what elements of spirituality are helpful to people growing out of adversity? Pargament describes what he terms the "critical ingredients of spirituality" (2006, 123) that are potentially related to growth: (1) support and empowerment, (2) meaning-making, and (3) fostering life-changing transformations of goals and priorities. What did our study participants have to say about spirituality and what they found helpful or meaningful while coping with difficult experiences? There were plenty of examples of ways in which spirituality provided some of the elements that Pargament talks about as key to how spirituality is associated with growth.

Sources of Strength, Support, and Empowerment

Some patients and physicians described their faith as their major source of strength during their experiences of difficulty. Darci put it this way:

> You can get through anything as long as you have the will and you've got faith and you've got people who love you. That was the thing that got me through—my family and my faith.

For some, that spiritual belief is a faith in a God that is a source of strength for them. Terri has had medical problems since childhood, suffering through many corrective surgeries. To her, God is a source of strength to get through the present, and a source of hope that things will not always be so difficult in the future.

> Has spirituality played a role? Definitely, it has. I know the pain psychologist asked me something along that line. I said I know that the Lord has helped me get through all this, so certainly he can help me the rest of the way. I have that confidence—sometimes it's a little

shaky—but it's a trust and faith, and I know I'm going to have a new body someday. There is a woman I know who was paralyzed in a diving accident, and I do listen to her. She's in a wheelchair, and yet she started a Wheelchairs around the World program to help children whose lives could benefit so much if they had wheelchairs and were able to get around. She shares the gospel. She will sing a song about not being able to do things here on Earth, but she knows she'll be able to do them in heaven. So that's encouraging—that being on this Earth isn't all there is.

Meaning in Suffering

There were also of examples of what Pargament and colleagues would put in the category of meaning-making, as participants described ways in which their faith helped them to give meaning to their situation. Dr. H struggled to understand the mistake that he was involved in as a young resident, a mistake that caused the death of a child.

> Spirituality has certainly been helpful, because part of that for me is having the faith that whatever happens, I can get through it. I will look back and I will be able to figure out what the meaning of all that was. Everything has a meaning or a purpose, and this is a testing or a trial or a path that I have to walk at this moment. It may not make sense to me now, but it's going to be okay.

One physician had grown up Catholic, but became Sufi. He put the mistakes in this context:

> Everything's connected, and there's this deep love and beauty every moment. Just because you make a mistake, that's so small compared to all that other stuff that's so beautiful. That kind of washes away small things because they don't really matter in the end. I grew up a Catholic, but became a Sufi by accident. If I had been a Catholic, I

think I probably would have responded the same way, recognizing that it was connected to something bigger than myself.

Major Life Transformation

For some, spirituality played a role in viewing their adversity as a major turning point in their lives. Some physicians and patients, previously agnostics or atheists, developed a deep spirituality in the context of this adversity, which was key to their positive coping and fostered a complete transformation of their lives.

Dr. J was a middle-aged general surgeon who had a terrible struggle after a devastating medical error that resulted in a patient's death in the operating room. Her negative coping strategies included drugs and alcohol, a story all too common among physicians and nonphysicians alike in the aftermath of a tragedy. At some point, she hit bottom. Prior to this she had been an agnostic. Now in recovery, she talks about the importance of her spiritual beliefs:

> Without faith—and I mean that broadly—in a plane or level that is so much more than we are, all of this is meaningless. So my advice would be to develop a sense of faith and put meaning to it.

Joe, discussed in chapter 7, was a champion kickboxer and highly successful real estate investor who developed chronic pain and got into drugs and alcohol to manage his pain. His situation quickly spun out of control, and he found himself at rock bottom, homeless and penniless. He was led into recovery through a newfound faith. He prays daily and memorizes Bible verses that give him guidance and strength. He plans to go back to finish college, and he spends many hours helping others who struggle to turn their lives around. He says that his spirituality is like AA is to drinking: "You know how they say AA ruins your drinking? Well, that's how spirituality is in my life now."

These two stories were perhaps the most dramatic turning-point stories related to a religious awakening in people who were not previously religious. Some people had a previously existing faith, but in the wake of their suffering, their spiritual beliefs became central to their lives and their healing in unanticipated ways. Darci, whom we met in chapter 7, was one of those. Her transformational experience involved a reawakening of previous faith that had lapsed, but in her suffering she found her way into a renewed and reconstituted faith that helped her through her difficult times.

> My lowest point was when I was wishing myself to die. That was my turning point, and I snapped out of it. I went back to church, and I started reading the Bible. I mean, I had always believed in God, but then I lost my faith totally at one point. I stopped going to church, but you don't have to have a building to pray to God. So I got my faith back, and with the help of God and my children, and just knowing I had to get through this, that gave me the strength to go on. I hope I never have to take too many pain pills again for the rest of my life.

Notably these stories were not, for the most part, solitary conversion experiences. They involved other people who were part of a supportive community or family that served as a conduit of the spiritual message. Jenny suffered from debilitating sciatica. She found healing in an unexpected time and place.

> The turning point was last July. I went to Wales with my mother and sister. My mother is Welsh, so it was a homecoming trip for her. For my sister and me, we could see Wales through our mother's eyes as she showed us where she grew up. It turned into a sort of pilgrimage to all these sacred sites in Wales. My sister had a book about them. They included cathedrals, but also places like tombs or special mountains where a man would sit and commune with angels, and there was a history about that. There were lots of places

where there were legends that something important happened on this site. A spring just came out of the earth and water appeared, and if you touch this water or anoint yourself with this water or immerse yourself in this water you will be healed.

Now I was going to every place and immersing my ankle into that water. At the last place we went to, there was a legend about a saint, and it was a big place with a big pool and lots and lots of people. A little museum in the front has hundreds of pairs of crutches where people have come and immersed themselves in the water and left their crutches behind. That has been going on for thousands of years. I decided, "I am going in." I didn't have a bathing suit, but I was going in. It felt a little awkward to take something that seriously and to put myself in that position, but I did. I immersed myself fully into the pool. But then a really powerful, meaningful thing happened afterward: my mother offered to give a prayer. My mother is a very spiritual person. She is an ordained Methodist minister, and it was so powerful to have her support and her power of prayer and intention and spirituality join mine in helping my back to heal. She poured some of the water onto my back and said a prayer. My mother is not an airy fairy. She is a no-nonsense kind of woman. So that was pretty powerful, and I would say that would be the turning point.

Dr. J, who had the most dramatic turnaround in relation to her experience of a devastating medical error, expressed that without some notion of something bigger than herself, it would have been much more difficult, perhaps impossible, to go on.

I'm convinced that spirituality got me through it to the point where I could finally function again. I was totally agnostic before this.

Dr. X, on the other hand, did not describe herself as spiritual. However, she noted the importance of spirituality in how her patient coped with the situation:

I'm not spiritual in a formal sense. But spirituality definitely is some part of how I think about things. I guess I would say that I think the patient was spiritual in how she accepted the situation. She made it fit into her spiritual view: *this is something that happened, and I have to live my life with this.* That had meaning for me. Spirituality fit in somehow, because I feel as if that's how she coped, and that resonated for me.

Doing the Right Thing: A Calling to a Better Self

Spirituality—whether religious or not—seemed to offer an important moral framework for helping some people in our study to do the right thing in these difficult circumstances. For those who were religious, the religious teachings, as well as the experience of grace, provided the guidance that helped them discern right action and the strength to carry it out. Remember Dr. C, who struggled to go back into her patient's room to apologize for her error? In her opinion, what helped her do the right thing was this concept of grace.

> The hardest thing of all was having to walk into that room to apologize. Not knowing what I was going to face, except knowing that I had to do that because it was the right thing to do. And I could only do that with grace. I wouldn't have had the power to do that myself because I felt ashamed, guilty, and afraid. To me, grace is what gave me the power to walk through that door, to face him and his family.

Interestingly, this grace was not just something to be received, but something that also propelled compassionate action toward others. In other words, the grace was not only vertical but horizontal and relational.

Alan Alfano, a rehabilitation physician, put it this way in the film *Choosing Wisdom*:

> It helps me to be humble and gracious when I think about how someone much greater than I has been gracious toward me.

Dr. D, though she did not describe herself as innately spiritual, was moved spiritually by a patient's extension of grace to her.

I guess from the spiritual standpoint, I was just so amazed with how gracious, how open and accepting he has been, just being able to have me still there. He must have blamed me. Who wouldn't? But that never came out. I feel as if his being able to let me stay involved was how I got through all of it.

Some physicians rejected the religious notions of spirituality, but did speak of a calling to the profession. With that calling came a sense of something larger than themselves, drawing them to a profession that involved subsuming their own needs and desires to those of their patients. This larger purpose for their role as doctors pulled them into a life of true service to others. The professional code of ethics, as well as a deeper sense of service, honor, and justice, compelled them to do the right thing in situations where their own self-interest would have had them do otherwise.

Dr. Alfano, the rehabilitation physician, describes it this way:

I decided that I should go over and talk with the patient, although everything in me just wanted to run the other way. In the end, that is not who we are as physicians. We care for the patient, even when— especially when—things have not gone well.

Dr. Alfano continued,

I really care about the people, and I really want to do something worthwhile for them. I want to be part of a solution, part of a healing process. That's what I am called to do. If that's the case, I have to be able to look beyond mistakes that I make to something that is bigger than me, which is the purpose that I am involved in.

Dr. V describes a mistake early in his career that he found particularly difficult because he felt it represented some hubris on his part as a young physician. Since that day he has taken to heart what he feels is a crucial part of the professional code, and that is checking your ego at the door.

> When it comes to patient care, you have to be willing to commit yourself wholly to it without ego, ask for help when it's appropriate, and be honest with yourself and with everybody else around you to try to make things better.

That has helped him do the right thing and prevented mistakes of hubris from occurring again. He also feels strongly that by facing his mistakes and doing something positive following his errors, he is able to honor the memory of the person he harmed, and achieve a kind of reconciliation.

> You need to find a way to externalize that, to deal with the stress, and then to figure out a way to move forward positively and to take that negative and make it something positive—whether it's just on a personal level, making sure that you personally don't make that same error again, or sharing it with other people or changing the culture and making things safer. If you can do something positive with that negative event, then it's not a waste. I tend to think of the Gettysburg Address: "That from these honored dead we take increased devotion." I think that is a way of moving forward from something like this.

This sense of calling to a profession of service helped these physicians overcome their own self-interest and set them on the path to wisdom.

FORGIVENESS

Other than relating the story of the error, forgiveness was the topic that generated the most distressing emotion in our interviews with physicians. For some, forgiveness was not something that they could imagine for themselves. As one physician said,

> See, that "forgiveness" word—I just don't know what that means. I know how to forgive other people, but I don't know what it means to forgive myself. I don't know what that means. That's a big issue. I think the universe is a pretty unforgiving place, so I don't seek much forgiveness.

In some of those cases, the patient or family had extended their forgiveness, but the physician couldn't accept it.

Forgiveness is an important element in moving through adversity. But for physicians and patients, forgiveness was complicated and difficult.

Forgiveness is a complex notion for the doctors, is often inextricably linked with justice or atonement. Some of the physicians' stories reflected "partial forgiveness," as they noted their concern that forgiveness somehow might lower their standards. They cited a tension between forgiving their error and maintaining their high standards for care, whether technical or moral. Dr. M, who missed a diagnosis in a very complex case, talks about holding back from forgiving herself as a means of ensuring that she will maintain her drive to always do better.

> The only forgiveness that I decided to give myself is partial, to this day. I keep that other unforgiven part as the pressure to keep doing better. I think maybe that is one of the reasons that, for me, the forgiveness thing is always a little bit difficult because I guess you can forgive, but not forget. I worry about that a little bit. If I am completely forgiven, I will forget and that's not good for me.

In some cases there was a clear difference in how the physicians felt about forgiveness of different types of error or different facets of an error. Charles Bosk, in his book *Forgive and Remember*, writes of his eighteen-month embedded observation of the culture of surgeons. He describes a fundamental distinction that surgeons make between what he calls "technical" and "moral" errors. Surgeons can forgive each other for technical errors, and the appropriate response to those errors is simply to understand how they occurred and to correct them. But moral errors are handled differently. Moral errors, he observes, are "a failure to route problems properly because of professional pride or the failure to confess error or admit shortcomings." As he puts it,

> Physicians do not expect the application of medical knowledge to be perfect. There will always be honest errors. However, physicians do expect perfect compliance with the norms of clinical responsibility. They see this compliance as their best defense and remedy for the honest and inevitable errors they will all occasionally make. (Bosk 1979, 180–81)

Dr. V felt he couldn't forgive himself fully:

> I don't know if I've ever really fully forgiven myself, but I feel like going back to that. Establishing a track record for excellence sort of allows me to look on that one anomaly with a kinder eye. If I was having an event like that once a week, I might be more concerned. But I don't know if I'll ever fully forgive myself because of the undercurrent of pride and hubris that was associated with it, which I think was unacceptable. I was too cocky. I've tried really hard to check my ego at the door since then. I never let it get into the patient care mix again because that is the unforgivable sin that I committed.

For the physicians, grace or forgiveness was generally accompanied by some kind of restorative action. In some cases, that action started with disclosure and apology. Dr. V reflected on his disclosure to the patient. Although he had disclosed the error, he had not been as direct as he would have liked, and in retrospect it could have been more restorative to their trust relationship had he been more direct.

It was helpful for me to speak to the patient. I wish I had done a more appropriate disclosure to him, because I think that would have gone a long way for me.

Disclosure and apology were helpful in two ways. First, they began a restoration of the relationship of trust that, in the minds of the physicians, was broken by the error. The patients put their trust in the physician to keep them safe (*Primum no nocere* [First, do no harm]), and disclosure and apology were the first steps in restoring the trust and the sacred relationship between doctor and patient.

Second, disclosure and apology opened the door to the possibility of forgiveness, though the doctors were careful to say that expecting forgiveness was not only unrealistic but inappropriate. That being said, the physicians expressed surprise and enormous gratitude when the patients offered their forgiveness. In the case of Dr. C, the long-standing doctor-patient relationship was severed for over a month before the restorative meeting took place. The follow-up conversation occurred one month after the event, in which the physician again apologized and asked for forgiveness (though she was not expecting it). That conversation was truly restorative and offered healing to the physician and the patient, both of whom were suffering not only from the error but from the broken relationship. This physician went on to care for the patient in the following years up to the present day. We don't know how the patient feels at this point, but the physician commented that she was convinced that the restored relationship also helped the patient to heal physically, as he has unexpectedly survived his cancer.

Restorative action went beyond disclosure and apology. Some exemplars described an almost zealous dedication to the process of understanding why the error had occurred and doing whatever it took to prevent that error from recurring. That step was essential to reconciliation, whether it was internal (just within the physician's own being) or relational (either between the physician and the patient, or between the physician and God).

Finally, forgiving themselves was very often accomplished in the context of the physicians finally accepting their humanity. One doctor described a situation that was not a mistake in her care of the patient; however, the patient irrationally felt that perhaps the doctors could have anticipated the heart attack he suffered more than a year after she had seen him for a routine checkup. She found it difficult to let go of blame, even years after, even though she knew that her self-blame was irrational. She describes her eventual self-forgiveness this way:

> I guess over time I forgave myself. I still wish I had gotten the EKG and I wish I had been lucky. It went from being a mistake to more like, well, this is what being human is like.

Justice, Forgiveness, and Spirituality

For many of the physicians, justice, forgiveness, and spirituality were inextricably intertwined. Some form of doing the right thing with regard to the patient was both required by and aided by their spiritual understanding of themselves and their place in the world. In this way, disclosure, apology, and forgiveness became a kind of relational reconciliation. If their spirituality had to do with their professional calling, then the professional code of honor helped them to do the honorable thing, despite their own feelings and even despite what lawyers may have told them they should not do in order to protect their self-interest.

If their spirituality was of a religious nature, the concepts of humility and grace were experienced as necessary for their own forgiveness, but also elements that then extended to right action—extending compassion, mercy, grace, and forgiveness to others.

Forgiveness in our study's patient population was, for most patients, focused on forgiving others. (The exception to this was in cases where there was an accident for which the patient felt responsible. In those cases self-forgiveness was considered by the patients to be difficult and important for positive growth.) It is interesting to note that many of the patients felt that forgiving others (or themselves) was important to being able to move forward in relation to their pain. Not being able to forgive someone was seen by some patients as a real roadblock to their healing. Barbara, who suffered with pain for years, put it this way:

Has forgiveness played a role? Oh, yes, definitely. You can't have grudges and hatreds and have a free spirit.

Patricia, who had pain so severe she could not sit up, hold a book, or sleep, found that forgiveness was key to her own recovery.

I guess I have benefited from a husband who is a psychologist. There have been a lot of books around and a lot of discussion. I had some really bad issues with my brother: we didn't have a relationship for about seven years. Then I started to realize that it doesn't hurt anyone but me, and I have forgiven my brother for a lot of what went on. Letting go of it felt very good, very life-affirming, and now I have a relationship with my brother that is positive.

Forgiveness was very hard for some patients, some of whom had suffered unspeakable abuses. But many patients found that letting go of those old grudges, and forgiving those who had wronged them, was very freeing and helped them to recover. Some, like Joe, cultivate this forgiveness into a daily practice:

I used to have resentments. There was someone who picked on me in seventh and eighth grade, and it really changed my life. I thought of him for years. When I exercised, I'd think of this kid's name when lifting weights. It was pretty sad. Forty years old and I'm still dwelling on this from the distant past. So now if I catch myself being mad at somebody, I'll stop and I'll pray for them—pray for God to bless them and hold them in his hand. That's kind of how I handle it.

For patients and doctors, spirituality and forgiveness were complex but powerful sources of strength and guidance as they moved forward through their experience of adversity. Their beliefs prompted them to take positive action, empowered them, and moved them toward restoration of themselves, their relationships, and their positive role in the world. For some, this represented transformative experiences and major turning points. For most, these were iterative experiences that built on one another, slowly restoring the self in positive relation to the world.

14. Choosing Wisdom

Between stimulus and response there is a space. In that space is our power to choose our response. In our response lies our growth and our freedom. —VICTOR FRANKL

Everything we have can be taken from us but one thing—the last of the human freedoms—to choose one's attitude in any given circumstance. —VICTOR FRANKL

Every time there are losses there are choices to be made. You choose to live your losses as passages to anger, blame, hatred, depression and resentment, or you choose to let these losses be passages to something new, something wider and deeper. —HENRI NOUWEN

MIDWAY THROUGH OUR ANALYSIS of the interview data, during a meeting of our research group, we were combing through some of the themes, comparing notes and looking for common threads. Suddenly, we all realized at nearly the same moment that one theme was strikingly common to all the exemplar stories: choice. Wisdom didn't just happen to these people. The path to wisdom was a series of choices—difficult, courageous, conscious, and intentional. This is not to imply that people knew exactly where these choices would lead them. In fact, the courage of these choices often had to do with the fact that the path was not at all clear. Choosing to step into the situation, to be open, to take responsibility, to try something different, to be honest— without knowing where things were leading—required courage. Some would say that situations of adversity are powerful precisely because they leave people with no choice, but that is not the case. The people in our study had no choice about their circumstance, but they had a choice about their response, which was all they needed for wisdom to grow. In that space that Frankl talks about, between our circumstance and our response to that circumstance, the seeds of wisdom are sown.

That choice was sometimes dramatic, a real turning point at a particular moment. For Dr. J, the turning point came in the middle of the night. She was at her absolute lowest point, completely unable to function as a wife, a mother, or a doctor after a devastating error. She had been trying to cope in negative and eventually self-destructive ways, turning to drugs and alcohol to dull her emotions. She woke up in the middle of the night, and realized she had a choice to make if she was going to get better.

For others, there were continuous and less dramatic choices that made a difference.

Henri Nouwen was a theologian and a respected teacher. Toward the end of his life he chose to move to Canada and live at L'Arche, where people with disabilities of many kinds live together in intentional community. He saw the extreme difficulties with which these people coped yet was impressed daily with their joy. "If I describe everybody's life in the physical, you would see a lot of pain, a lot of struggle, a lot of difficulty. But somehow it's a very joyful community, because they've all chosen to live in a certain way, to live their pain in a certain way" (Nouwen 2007). He goes on to talk about how these are not singular choices, but ones we make and remake every day. "We make a lot of mistakes. It's not like once and forever; we are constantly invited again to choose. I know it for myself. I have to keep choosing . . . to say 'yes,' 'yes,' and 'yes' yet again" (Nouwen 2007).

Maurice, a military veteran, described the continual choice between focusing on joy or pain.

> You make a decision. You can either stay in this area of pain, or you can say, "You know what, pain? *Sayonara*, I'm out of here. I'm going back to joy." But pain is always going to be around.

When a doctor chooses to go into the room each morning and talk with the patient she's harmed, rather than sending in the resident, she takes a step closer to reestablishing relationship and reconciliation.

When patients choose to explore ways in which they can use the interaction between mind and body to help them cope with pain, each attempt opens up new possibilities. They are now actively exploring and learning, and choices that build on themselves.

When physicians choose to be honest and open about a mistake, an opportunity opens up for learning (*how did that happen and how can we prevent it from happening again?*), as well as the opportunity for reestablishing trust with the patient.

Sharon was injured in a motor vehicle accident. She experiences pain every day, but she describes making the choice every day for life. On the bad days, it comes down to perseverance:

> I think it has to do with perseverance. Today may seem bad, but tomorrow you may wake up and the pain will be gone.... Whatever it is—you have to have something within your domain that you look forward to tomorrow.

When asked what helped them to move through these experiences in a positive way, community was the most all-encompassing. In community, people were first of all able to see that they were not alone on this journey, that the journey of suffering is universal; only the form of suffering changes. In community, others who had suffered similar circumstances were eager to share what they had learned, and that sharing was indeed part of their healing. People's suffering, if they moved through it positively, softened them, made them more forgiving and more compassionate, and helping another became an almost irresistible act. It is as though this experience is hardwired to bring us together if approached in a positive way. And it makes me wonder if indeed it is possible as a culture to embrace and foster the capacities for wisdom as we inch closer to embodying it fully.

One thing appears to be true from our study: adversity is an opportunity for the development of wisdom. That is not to say that it is the only opportunity for wisdom, but it seems that the breaking open of our more comfortable way of being is the fertile ground in which the seeds of wisdom are sown. However, once we are sensitized by a situation of suffering and become aware of, or get a taste of, the capacity for wisdom, we can and do continue to grow by fostering that awareness. By noticing and attending to the suffering of others, we expand our capacity for compassion. By appreciating the beauty around us and being aware of our place in the wider creation, we expand our ability to see the bigger picture, less driven by our own needs. By reflecting on our own actions and actively trying to see things from many perspectives, we begin to build our capacity to tolerate complexity and ambiguity and avoid black-and-white thinking. In other words, we can "practice" wisdom.

These points inevitably lead to the question of whether, as a parent, teacher, or community we can "teach" wisdom. I think we already try to do just that, in small ways, through storytelling. If you are a parent, think about the stories you tell your children. Many of them have a message—a little bit of wisdom that you want to share with your children so that they don't have to go through what you, or your uncle Jack, or your parents went through. Those wisdom stories seem to intensify as your children get to the age of leaving the nest, when the urge to do a wisdom dump directly into your children's hard drive becomes almost irresistible. Of course, much of that wisdom seems to fall on deaf ears, until an experience of their own resonates with that story and which then begins to have meaning for them. Medical practitioners do a similar thing, but some stories are missing. As we heard from our physician participants, the stories of mistakes are absent from the culture of medicine. Instead, a myth of the perfect physician is perpetuated, perhaps unintentionally but quite powerfully, and not only within medicine but among the public. With that myth comes another: that as humans we are in complete control of our bodies—that we can put off death and illness indefinitely, that we can conquer all that threatens us.

The myth is seductive and powerful, but it is the antithesis of wisdom.

What would it be like if we trained doctors with the explicit intention of developing their capacity for wisdom? As a counterbalance to knowledge acquisition and the honing of skills, medical schools would also intentionally foster a keen sense of the complex and ambiguous nature of the decisions we must make, an awareness of our own vulnerability, careful attention to the bigger picture, and the capacity to see things from many perspectives. What if we chose students for their capacity for self-reflection, compassion, and their tolerance for ambiguity rather than, or in addition to, their scores on the Medical College Admissions Test? Wisdom researcher Robert Sternberg is investigating ways to supplement the traditional MCAT in the selection of medical students that better predict success in medical school (2008).

Training physicians, though, is just a microcosm of society at large, and it is interesting to ask whether a community that intentionally begins to cultivate the capacity for wisdom might be able to achieve a higher level of harmony and flourishing. Is there such a thing as a wise organization or community? Are we ready for wisdom on a large scale?

The good news is that we do indeed have a choice, not about the hand that life deals us, but in the way that we play the hand. And it appears from our study that how we deal with that circumstance has the potential to change our lives (and perhaps other people's lives) for the better.

I realized that I had a choice. I could choose to stay in that dark place, blaming myself and feeling as if life isn't really worth living, or I could choose to get out of it, and use that situation for the betterment of the world.

Questions for Reflection and Discussion

Part One: Background

Chapter 1: Introduction

The authors of this book hope that others will begin to develop curiosity about wisdom. What attracted you to this book? What do you hope to learn or gain by reading it?

Do you have any personal stories of wisdom that you will reflect on as you read this book and the stories in it?

What qualities do you think are most important for us to cultivate throughout our lives? Is wisdom one of those qualities? Why or why not?

Chapter 2: Defining Wisdom

How would you define "wisdom"? How does your definition compare to the dictionary definitions?

Why is wisdom important, and why do we aspire to be wise?

Describe one of the wisest people you know. What about that person makes you feel he or she is wise?

Do you have an example of wisdom in action?

How do we share wisdom (as teachers, parents, or friends)?

Do you think that ordinary people can be wise? Is it possible to be wise one minute and not wise the next?

Chapter 3: Posttraumatic Growth

Think about a difficult circumstance that you have faced. How did you change in a positive way because of this circumstance? What did you learn about yourself?

What helped you move through this circumstance in a positive way?

Have you changed how you think about or do things, or have your priorities shifted because of this difficulty that you faced?

How do you think you can help others who face difficulty in their lives? What advice would you give them, knowing what you know now?

Part Two: The Path through Adversity

Chapter 4: Acceptance

Can you describe a time when you moved from denial to acceptance? How long did it take? How did you feel?

What specifically helped you accept that difficult circumstance? Have you ever helped someone else become more accepting?

Did you change in other ways when you became more accepting?

Chapter 5: Stepping In

How would you describe this notion of "stepping in"? What different types of stepping in did we see in this chapter?

Why is stepping in an important element of wisdom development? Can you be a wise person without taking responsibility for your actions?

Dr. C failed to diagnose her patient's lung cancer, and her patient was very upset with her. Later she went to his hospital room, and he accepted her apology. How would you have reacted if you had been her patient in that situation?

Can you think of a time when you needed to step in to a situation, even though it was difficult? Did you do it? What was the result?

The physicians in this and other chapters talk a lot about the shame of making a mistake. Do you think that they should feel shame? Why or why not?

If a doctor makes a serious error, what can he or she do to mitigate that error? How does this relate to wisdom development?

Chapter 6: Integration

Think about a difficult experience in your life, one that challenged your understanding of the world or yourself. How did you integrate that experience into your life? How did your understanding of the world or of yourself have to change?

What helped you to integrate this experience successfully?

Chapter 7: New Narrative

Think of something that happened to you today—something you did or something someone said to you—that you have woven into your personal narrative. Was it a positive thread or a negative thread?

Did you say or do something to others today that they could weave into their narrative? Did you tell a student that she was an excellent writer? Did you listen to your son practice his guitar? How did you have an impact on others' understanding of themselves today?

This chapter was about taking lessons that people learned from one experience (error or pain) and applying it to a new experience (family, illness, medicine). Why is this important? If we don't apply lessons to new situations, what happens?

This chapter was also about making changes, including becoming stronger and more compassionate. Are there other ways to learn these lessons, or do they have to be learned through adversity?

Think of something important that you learned in one situation that you have been able to apply to another. Perhaps you learned a lesson in childhood that you carry with you today.

Reframing is a marvelous technique that anyone can do. Think of something that seems like a negative in your life today—big or small—and try your hand at reframing. What is another way to look at this situation? How can you reframe this particular problem into something beneficial or positive?

Chapter 8: Wisdom

If you could give your children a life free of tragedy and pain, would you? Why or why not?

Think about someone, and it could be yourself, who has suffered an unimaginable tragedy but who seems to have grown from the experience. Describe this person. Why do you think he or she has grown? How can you tell? How do you feel when you think about this person?

Are people who grow as a result of tragedy different from most people? Different from you? In what ways?

Some wonderful characters in literature have chosen wisdom in the midst of adversity. Who is your favorite, and what did that character experience?

PART THREE: WHAT HELPS? SAGE ADVICE FROM THE FIELD

Chapter 9: Finding Community

This chapter talks a lot about the importance of sharing stories. In what ways is story sharing an important part of our lives, not only in the instance of tragedy?

Imagine going through an entire day without sharing or hearing a single story. What would that day be like? How would you feel?

Several examples appear in this chapter of people feeling immensely better after sharing their story with a group of trusted people. Why do you think this opportunity to share has such a profound effect on people who are suffering?

Can you think of people who are suffering who are unable to participate in supportive communities? What about these people prevents them from joining a community?

Do you need to talk things through when you're troubled? How does that help you? Whom do you talk to about your problems?

What if you're a person who is not comfortable sharing personal information or stories with others? In what other ways could you integrate emotions, as Pennebaker and Seagal suggest?

If something terrible happened to you today, what community would you turn to for help and comfort? How would these people be able to help you?

In what ways do you provide a listening ear to people who are suffering?

Why might a role model for healing be important to someone who is suffering? Have you ever experienced a tragedy and looked to someone else as an example of how to survive?

Where would someone go to find a role model for healing?

Chapter 10: Gratitude and Compassion

Have you cultivated a practice of gratitude? Name five things you are grateful for today.

Have you ever experienced a shift from irritation or another negative reaction to compassion?

When you are in a bad mood, what do you do to shift to a more positive outlook?

Chapter 11: Quiet Reflection, Meditation, and Mindfulness

What are some ways you bring the relaxation response into your life? Have there been times when you became particularly aware of the connection between stress, relaxation, and well-being?

Do you meditate? If so, has your practice changed your life? In what ways?

Describe what "mindfulness" means to you and a time when mindfulness may have given you insight into a difficult life circumstance.

Chapter 12: Doing Something

Neuroscientist Adele Diamond tells her son to "just do your homework" and be transformed in the process. What does she mean? How can you be transformed by doing something that you don't really want to do? What is necessary for this transformation to occur?

To some, this chapter may sound a bit Pollyannaish. Do you think that some pain may be too severe, that "just doing something" is a rather simplistic piece of advice? Why do you think that?

Do you know someone who has done something creative or interesting to cope with adversity? What did this person do? Did it seem to help? Why?

List one activity that you do now that truly brings you joy and pleasure. Imagine if you could no longer do this activity because of an injury or some other event. How would you cope? What would you do instead?

Chapter 13: Spirituality, Forgiveness, and Doing the Right Thing

Would you describe yourself as a spiritual person? If so, has that spirituality been helpful to you in difficult times? Have life's difficulties presented challenges to your spirituality?

What helps you do the right thing in difficult circumstances?

Are there times in your life when forgiveness helped you heal from a difficult circumstance?

Are there people whom you have difficulty forgiving? Are there things that you have done for which you have not forgiven yourself? How do you think that affects you?

Chapter 14: Choosing Wisdom

Think of some situation in your life right now in which you have an opportunity to choose wisdom.

How can you foster wisdom in your life? What disciplines do you think would help you grow in wisdom?

References

Part One

Proust, M. 1919. *In Search of Lost Time*. Vol. 2: *Within a Budding Grove*.

Rumi. 1995. *The Essential Rumi*. Trans. Coleman Barks. San Francisco: HarperSanFrancisco.

Chapter 1

Calhoun, L., and R. Tedeschi, eds. 2006. *Handbook of Posttraumatic Growth*. New York: Lawrence Erlbaum Associates.

Haidt, J. 2006. *The Happiness Hypothesis*. New York: Basic Books.

Hall, S. 2010. *Wisdom: From Philosophy to Neuroscience*. New York: Random House.

Nietzsche, F. 1997/1889. *Twilight of the Idols*. Indianapolis: Hackett.

Remen, R. 1996. *Kitchen Table Wisdom*. New York: Riverhead Books.

Chapter 2

Achenbaum, A. W., and L. Orwoll. 1991. "Becoming Wise: A Psycho-Gerontological Interpretation of the Book of Job." *International Journal of Aging and Human Development* 32: 21–39.

Alter, R. 2010. *The Wisdom Books: Job, Proverbs and Ecclesiastes*. New York: Norton & Company.

Ardelt, M. 2000a. "Antecedents and Effects of Wisdom in Old Age: A Longitudinal Perspective on Aging Well." *Research on Aging* 22(4): 360–94.

———. 2000b. "Intellectual versus Wisdom-Related Knowledge: The Case for a Different Kind of Learning in the Later Years of Life." *Educational Gerontology* 26: 771–89.

———. 2003. "Empirical Assessment of a Three-Dimensional Wisdom Scale." *Research on Aging* 25(3): 275–324.

———. 2004. "Wisdom as Expert Knowledge System: A Critical Review of a Contemporary Operationalization of an Ancient Concept." *Human Development* 47: 257–85.

———. 2005. "How Wise People Cope with Crises and Obstacles in Life." *ReVision* 28: 7–19.

Aristotle. 1924. *Metaphysics*. Trans. W. D. Ross. Oxford: Oxford University Press.

———. 1954. *Nichomachean Ethics I*. Trans. W. D. Ross. Oxford: Clarendon Press.

Baltes, P. B., and J. Smith. 1990. "Towards a Psychology of Wisdom and Its Ontogenesis." In *Wisdom: Its Nature, Origins, and Development*, ed. R. J. Sternberg, 87–120. Cambridge: Cambridge University Press.

Bluck, S., and J. Gluck. 2004. "Making Things Better and Learning a Lesson: Experiencing Wisdom across the Lifespan." *Journal of Personality* 72(1): 1–19.

Cantwell, C. 2010. *Buddhism: The Basics*. NY: Routledge.

Clayton, V. 1982. "Wisdom and Intelligence: The Nature and Function of Knowledge in the Later Years." *International Journal on Aging and Development* 15: 315–23.

———, and J. Birren. 1980. "The Development of Wisdom across the Life Span: A Re-Examination of an Ancient Topic." In *Life Span Development and Behavior*, vol. 3, ed. Paul Baltes and Orville G. Brim Jr.: 103–35. New York: Academic Press.

Erikson, E. 1950. *Childhood and Society*. New York: Norton.

Gluck, J., S. Bluck, J. Baron, and D. P. McAdams. 2005. "The Wisdom of Experience: Autobiographical Narratives across Adulthood." *International Journal of Behavioral Development* 29(3): 197–208.

———. 2007. "Looking Back across the Life Span: A Life Story Account of the Reminiscence Bump." *Memory & Cognition* 35(8): 1928–39.

———. 2011. "Laypeople's Conceptions of Wisdom and Its Development: Cognitive and Integrative Views." *The Journal of Gerontology, Series B: Psychological Sciences and Social Sciences* 66(3): 321–24.

Joseph, S., and P. A. Linley. 2006. "Growth Following Adversity: Theoretical Perspectives and Implications for Clinical Practice." *Clinical Psychology Review* 26: 1041–53.

Pascual-Leone, J. 2000. "Mental Attention, Consciousness, and the Progressive Emergence of Wisdom." *Journal of Adult Development* 7(4): 241–54.

Pennebaker, J. W. 2000. "Telling Stories: The Health Benefits of Narrative." *Literature and Medicine* 19(1): 3–18.

———, and J. D. Seagal. 1999. "Forming a Story: The Health Benefits of Narrative." *Journal of Clinical Psychology* 55(10): 1243–54.

Plato. 1950. *Dialogues of Plato (The Jowett Translations)*. Ed. J. Kaplan. New York: Simon and Schuster.

———. 1969. *Plato: The Last Days of Socrates*. Trans. H. Tredennick. Middlesex, UK: Penguin Books.

Remen, R. 1996. *Kitchen Table Wisdom*. New York: Riverhead Books.

Rilke, R. M. 2001. *Letters to a Young Poet*. New York: Random House.

Robinson, D. N. 1990. Wisdom through the Ages. In *Wisdom: Its Nature, Origins, and Development*, ed. R. Sternberg, 13–24. Cambridge: Cambridge University Press.

Staudinger, U. and Gluck J. 2011. "Psychological Wisdom Research: Commonalities and Differences in a Growing Field." *Annual Review of Psychology* 62: 215–41.

Sternberg, R. 1990. "Wisdom and Its Relations to Intelligence and Creativity." In *Wisdom: Its Nature, Origins, and Development*, ed. R. Sternberg, 142–60. Cambridge: Cambridge University Press.

———. 2004. "What Is Wisdom and How Can We Develop It?" *The Annals of the American Academy of Political and Social Science* 591: 164–74.

Strong, J. 2001. *Buddha: A Short Biography*. Oxford: Oneworld.

Wallis, G. 2007. *Basic Teachings of the Buddha*. New York: Random House.

———. 2007. *The Dhammapada: Verses on the Way*. New York: Random House.

Internet Resources

The Wisdom Page: http://www.wisdompage.com/index.html

Collective Wisdom Initiative: http://www.collectivewisdominitiative.org/

Defining Wisdom: http://wisdomresearch.org/

Chapter 3

Baltes, P. B., and J. Smith. 1990. "Towards a Psychology of Wisdom and Its Ontogenesis." In *Wisdom: Its Nature, Origins, and Development*, ed. R. J. Sternberg, 87–120. Cambridge: Cambridge University Press.

Bell, R. H. 2007. *Rethinking Justice: Restoring Our Humanity*. Lanham, MD: Lexington Books.

Bower, J. E., M. E. Kemeny, S. E. Tylor, and J. L. Fahey. 1998. "Cognitive Processing, Discovery of Meaning, CD 4 Decline, and AIDS-Related

Mortality among Bereaved HIV-Seropositive Men." *Journal of Consulting and Clinical Psychology* 66: 979–86.

Calhoun, L., A. Cann, R. Tedeschi, and J. McMillan. 2000. "A Correlational Test of the Relationship between Posttraumatic Growth, Religion, and Cognitive Processing." *Journal of Traumatic Stress* 13: 521–27.

Calhoun, L., and R. Tedeschi. 2004. "Foundations of Posttraumatic Growth: New Considerations." *Psychological Inquiry* 15(1): 93–102.

———, eds. 2006. *Handbook of Posttraumatic Growth*. New York: Lawrence Erlbaum Associates.

Cann, A., L. Calhoun, R. Tedeschi, and D. T. Solomon. 2010. "Posttraumatic Growth and Depreciation as Independent Experiences and Predictors of Well-Being." *Journal of Loss and Trauma* 15(3): 151–66.

Charon, R. 2006. *Narrative Medicine: Honoring the Stories of Illness*. New York: Oxford University Press.

Clark, L. 1996. "Restructuring and Realigning Mental Models: Ruminations as Guides to Cognitive Home Repair." In *Ruminative Thoughts: Advances in Social Cognition,* vol. 9, ed. R. S. Wyer, 63–72. New Jersey: Lawrence Erlbaum Associates.

Hefferon, K., M. Grealy, and N. Mutrie. 2009. "Posttraumatic Growth and Life-Threatening Physical Illness: A Systematic Review of the Qualitative Literature." *British Journal of Health Psychology* 14: 343–78.

Janoff-Bulman, R. 2006. "Schema-Change Perspectives on Posttraumatic Growth." In *Handbook of Posttraumatic Growth: Research and Practice,* ed. L. Calhoun and R. Tedeschi, 81–99. New York: Lawrence Erlbaum Associates.

Kierkegaard, S. 1938. *Purity of Heart Is to Will One Thing*. New York: Harper & Row.

Lerner, M. 2010. *Responses to Victimization and Belief in a Just World*. New York: Plenum Press.

Lewis, C. S. 1961. *A Grief Observed*. New York: Seabury Press.

Linley, P. A., and S. Joseph. 2004. "Positive Change Following Trauma and Adversity: A Review." *Journal of Traumatic Stress*: 17(1); 11–21.

Martin, L., and A Tesser. 1996. "Some Ruminative Thoughts" and "Clarifying Our Thoughts." In *Ruminative Thoughts: Advances in Social Cognition,* vol. 9, ed R. S. Wyer, 1–49 and 189–209. Hillsale, NJ: Lawrence Erlbaum Associates.

Neimeyer, R. 2006. "Re-Storying Loss: Fostering Growth in the Posttraumatic Narrative." In *Handbook of Posttraumatic Growth: Research and Practice,* ed. L. Calhoun and R. Tedeschi, 68–80. New York: Lawrence Erlbaum Associates.

Nietzsche, F. 1997/1889. *Twilight of the Idols.* Indianapolis: Hackett.

Pargament, K., K. Desai, and K. McConnel. 2006. "Spirituality: A Pathway to Posttraumatic Growth or Decline?" In *Handbook of Posttraumatic Growth: Research and Practice,* ed. L. Calhoun and R. Tedeschi, 121–37. New York: Larwrence Erlbaum Associates.

Park, C., C. Aldwin, J. Fenster, and L. Snyder. 2008. "Pathways to Posttraumatic Growth Versus Posttraumatic Stress: Coping and Emotional Reactions Following the September 11, 2001, Terrorist Attacks." *American Journal of Orthopsychiatry* 78(3): 300–12.

Pennebaker, J. W. 2000. "Telling Stories: The Health Benefits of Narrative." *Literature and Medicine* 19(1): 3–18.

———, and J. Seasac. 1999. "Forming a Story: The Health Benefits of Narrative." *Journal of Clinical Psychology* 55(10): 1243–54.

Remen, R. 1996. *Kitchen Table Wisdom.* New York: Riverhead Books.

Salik, E., and C. Auerbach. 2006. "From Devastation to Integration: Adjusting to and Growing from Medical Trauma." *Qualitative Health Research* 16(8): 1021–37.

Tait, R., and R. C. Silver. 1989. "Coming to Terms with Major Negative Life Events." In *Unintended Thought,* ed. J. S. Uleman and J. A. Barg, 351–82. New York: Guilford.

Tedeschi, R., and L. Calhoun. 1995. *Trauma and Transformation: Growing in the Aftermath of Suffering.* Thousand Oaks, CA: Sage Publications.

———. 1996. "The Posttraumatic Growth Inventory: Measuring the Positive Legacy of Trauma." *Journal of Traumatic Stress* 9: 455–71.

———. 2004. "Posttraumatic Growth: Conceptual Foundations of Empirical Evidence." *Psychological Inquiry* 15(1): 1–18.

Chapter 4

Achenbaum, W. A. 2004. "Wisdom's Vision of Relations." *Human Development* 47(5): 300–303.

Becker, E. 1997. *The Denial of Death.* New York: Free Press.

Greeson, J., J. Brantley, and F. Didonna. 2009. "Mindfulness and Anxiety Disorders: Developing a Wise Relationship with the Inner Experience of Fear." In *Clinical Handbook of Mindfulness*, ed. F. Didonna, 171–88. New York: Springer.

Lazarus, R. S. 2006. "Emotions and Interpersonal Relationships: Toward a Person-Centered Conceptualization of Emotions and Coping." *Journal of Personality* 74(1): 9–46.

Rogers, C. R. 1961. *On Becoming a Person: A Therapist's View of Psychotherapy*. Boston: Houghton Mifflin.

Chapter 5

Park, C., C. Aldwin, J. Fenster, and L. Snyder. 2008. "Pathways to Posttraumatic Growth versus Posttraumatic Stress: Coping and Emotional Reactions Following the September 11, 2001, Terrorist Attacks." *American Journal of Orthopsychology* 78(3): 300–312.

Perczek, R. E., M. A. Burke, C. S. Carver, A. Krongrad, and M. K. Terris. 2002. "Facing a Prostate Cancer Diagnosis." *Cancer* 94: 2923–29.

Silver, R. C., E. A. Holman, D. N. McIntosh, M. Poulin, and V. Gil-Rivas. 2002. "Nationwide Longitudinal Study of Psychological Responses to September 11." *JAMA* 288: 1235–44.

Turner, D., and H. Cox. 2004. "Facilitating Posttraumatic Growth." *Health and Quality of Life Outcomes* 2(34).

Chapter 6

Berlinger, N. 2005. *After Harm: Medical Error and the Ethics of Forgiveness*. Baltimore: Johns Hopkins University Press.

Bosk, C. 1979. *Forgive and Remember: Managing Medical Failure*. Chicago: University of Chicago Press.

Hilfiker, D. 1984. "Facing Our Mistakes." *New England Journal of Medicine* 310: 118–22.

———. 1998. *Healing the Wounds: A Physician Looks at His Work*. New York: Creighton University Press.

Neimeyer, R. 2006. "Re-Storying Loss: Fostering Growth in the Posttraumatic Narrative." In *Handbook of Posttraumatic Growth: Research and Practice*, ed. L. Calhoun and R. Tedeschi, 68–80. New York: Lawrence Erlbaum Associates.

Salick, E., and C. Auerbach. 2006. "From Devastation to Integration: Adjusting to and Growing from Medical Trauma." *Qualitative Health Research* 16(8): 1021–37.

Chapter 7

"A Woman's Burden." 2003. *Time.* March 28. http://www.time.com/time /nation/article/0,8599,438760,00.html#ixzz1ZC6DTvHi.

Cornum, R. 1993. *She Went to War: The Rhonda Cornum Story.* Novato, CA: Presidio Press.

Neimeyer, R. 2006. "Re-Storying Loss: Fostering Growth in the Posttraumatic Narrative." In *Handbook of Posttraumatic Growth: Research and Practice,* ed. L. Calhoun and R. Tedeschi, 68–80. New York: Lawrence Erlbaum Associates.

Orr, G. 2004. *The Blessing: A Memoir.* San Francisco: Council Oak Books.

Seligman, M. 2011. *Flourish: A Visionary New Understanding of Happiness and Well-Being.* New York: Free Press.

Spiegel, A. 2011. "For the Dying: A Chance to Rewrite Life." *Morning Edition.* NPR News. September 12.

Tedeschi, R., and L. Calhoun. 1995. *Trauma and Transformation: Growing in the Aftermath of Suffering.* Thousand Oaks, CA: Sage Publications.

———. 2004. "Posttraumatic Growth: Conceptual Foundations of Empirical Evidence." *Psychological Inquiry* 15(1): 1–18.

Tippett, Krista. 2010. "The Body's Grace: Matthew Sanford's Story." *Speaking of Faith.* American Public Media.

Chapter 8

Ardelt, M. 2003. "Empirical Assessment of a Three-Dimensional Wisdom Scale." *Research on Aging* 25(3): 275–324.

Baltes, P. B., and J. Smith. 1990. "Towards a Psychology of Wisdom and Its Ontogenesis." In *Wisdom: Its Nature, Origins, and Development,* ed. R. J. Sternberg, 87–120. Cambridge: Cambridge University Press.

Hall, S. 2010. *Wisdom: From Philosophy to Neuroscience.* New York: Random House.

Meacham J., 1990. "The Loss of Wisdom." In *Wisdom: Its Nature, Origins, and Development,* ed. R. J. Sternberg, 181–212. Cambridge: Cambridge University Press.

Nouwen, H. 1970. *Wounded Healer.* New York: Doubleday.

———. 1982. *Compassion.* New York: Doubleday.

Sternberg, R. 1990. "Wisdom and Its Relations to Intelligence and Creativity." In *Wisdom: Its Nature, Origins, and Development,* ed. R. J. Sternberg, 142–60. Cambridge: Cambridge University Press.

————. 1998. "A Balance Theory of Wisdom." *Reviews of General Psychology* 2(4); 347–65.

Suzuki, S. 2006. *Zen Mind, Beginner's Mind: Informal Talks on Meditation and Practice.* Boston: Shambhala Publications.

Chapter 9

Faces on Faith: Classic Interviews with 20th-Century Leaders (Desmond Tutu, Parker Palmer, and Adele Gonzales). 2008. EcuFilm distributed by Abingdon Press. Produced by United Methodist Communications and the Parish of Trinity Church/NYC.

Lown, B. A., and C. F. Manning. 2010. "The Schwartz Center Rounds: Evaluation of an Interdisciplinary Approach to Enhancing Patient-Centered Communication, Teamwork, and Provider Support." *Academic Medicine* 85(6): 1073–81.

Neimeyer, R. 2006. "Re-Storying Loss: Fostering Growth in the Posttraumatic Narrative." In *Handbook of Posttraumatic Growth: Research and Practice,* ed. L. Calhoun and R. Tedeschi, 140–60. New York: Lawrence Erlbaum Associates.

Orr, G. 2006. "This I Believe." *All Things Considered.* National Public Radio. February 20. Independently produced for NPR by Jay Allison and Dan Gediman with John Gregory and Viki Merrick.

Pennebaker, J. W., and J. D. Seagal. 1999. "Forming a Story: The Health Benefits of Narrative." *Journal of Clinical Psychology* 55(10): 1243–54.

Remen, R. N. 1996. *Kitchen Table Wisdom: Stories That Heal.* New York: Riverhead Books.

————. 2000. "From Zen Hospice." www.ijourney.org. May 29.

Salick, E. C., and C. F. Auerbach. 2006. "From Devastation to Integration: Adjusting to and Growing from Medical Trauma." *Qualitative Health Research* 16(8): 1021–37.

Sautter, U. 2010. "Reading, Writing, and Revelation." *ODE Magazine.* October. http://www.odemagazine.com.

Seligman, M. 2011. *Flourish: A Visionary New Understanding of Happiness and Well-Being.* New York: Free Press.

Strauss, D. 2010. *Half a Life: A Memoir.* New York: Random House.

Tedeschi, R. G., and L. G. Calhoun. 2004. "Posttraumatic Growth: Conceptual Foundations and Empirical Evidence." *Psychological Inquiry* 15(1): 1–18.

Von Hugel, Friedrich. 2001. *Letters to a Niece*. Vancouver: Regent College Publishing.

Chapter 10

Cicero, M. T. 1894. *The Orations of Marcus Tullius Cicero*. Vol. 3. London: G. Bell.

Dalai Lama. 2011. "The Transformation of Pain." November 5. http://www .dalailama.com.

Dickens, C. 1907. *David Copperfield*. London: Dent.

Emmons, R. A., and M. E. McCullough. 2003. "Counting Blessings versus Burdens: An Experimental Investigation of Gratitude and Subjective Well-Being in Daily Life." *Journal of Personality and Social Psychology* 84(2): 377–89.

Peterson, C. 2004. *Character Strengths and Virtues: A Handbook and Classification*. Washington, DC: American Psychological Association.

Seligman, M. 2011. *Flourish: A Visionary New Understanding of Happiness and Well-Being*. New York: Free Press.

Chapter 11

Baer, R. A. 2003. "Mindfulness Training as a Clinical Intervention: A Conceptual and Empirical Review." *Clinical Psychology: Science and Practice* 10(2): 125–43.

Benson, H. 1979. *The Mind/Body Effect: How Behavioral Medicine Can Show You the Way to Better Health*. New York: Simon and Schuster.

———. 1997. "The Relaxation Response: Therapeutic Effect." *Science* 278 (5344): 1693–97.

Bishop, S. R., M. Lau, S. Shapiro, L. Carlson, N. D. Anderson, J. Carmody, Z. V. Segal, S. Abbey, M. Speca, D. Velting, and G. Devins. 2004. "Mindfulness: A Proposed Operational Definition." *Clinical Psychology: Science and Practice* 11(3): 230–41.

Diamond, D. M. "Cognitive, Endocrine, and Mechanistic Perspectives on Non-Linear Relationships between Arousal and Brain Function." *Nonlinearity in Biology, Toxicology and Medicine* 3(1): 1–7.

Emerson, R. W. 1909. *Education, an Essay, and Other Selections*. Boston: Houghton Mifflin.

Five Masters of Meditation. 2002. Hartley Film Foundation.

Hanson, R., and R. Mendius. 2009. *Buddha's Brain: The Practical Neuro-*

science of Happiness, Love, and Wisdom. Oakland, CA: New Harbinger Publications.

Kabat-Zinn, J. 2003. "Mindfulness-Based Interventions in Context: Past, Present, and Future." *Clinical Psychology: Science and Practice* 10(2): 144–56.

———. 2010. *Mindfulness Meditation for Pain Relief: Guided Practices for Reclaiming Your Body and Your Life.* Boulder, CO: Sounds True.

Lutz, A., L. L. Greischar, N. B. Rawlings, M. Ricard, and R. J. Davidson. 2004. "Long-Term Meditators Self-Induce High-Amplitude Gamma Synchrony during Mental Practice." *Proceedings of the National Academy of Sciences of the United States of America* 101(46): 16369–73.

———. H. A. Slagter, J. D. Dunne, and R. J. Davidson. 2008. "Attention Regulation and Monitoring in Meditation." *Trends in Cognitive Sciences* 12(4): 163–69.

Marcus Aurelius. 1890. *The Meditations of Marcus Aurelius.* New York: Mershon Company.

Plews-Ogan, M., J. E. Owens, M. Goodman, P. Wolfe, and J. Schorling. 2005. "A Pilot Study Evaluating Mindfulness-based Stress Reduction and Massage for the Management of Chronic Pain." *Journal of General Internal Medicine* 20(12), 1136–38.

Raffone, A., and N. Srinivasan. "The Exploration of Meditation in the Neuroscience of Attention and Consciousness." *Cognitive Processing* 11(1): 1–7.

Raichle, M. E. 2010. "The Brain's Dark Energy." *Scientific American* 302(3): 44–49.

Travis, F., D. Haaga, J. Hagelin, M. Tanner, A. Arenander, S. Nidich, C. Gaylord-King, S. Grosswald, M. Rainforth, and R. Schneider. 2010. "A Self-Referential Default Brain State: Patterns of Coherence, Power, and eLORETA Sources during Eyes-Closed Rest and Transcendental Meditation Practice." *Cognitive Processing* 11(1): 21–30.

Treadway, M. T., S. W. Lazar, and F. Didonna. 2009. "The Neurobiology of Mindfulness." In *Clinical Handbook of Mindfulness,* ed. F. Didonna, 45–57. New York: Springer.

Chapter 12

Diamond, A. 2009. "Learning, Doing, Being: A New Science of Education." Interview on *Krista Tippitt on Being.* American Public Media. November 19. http://being.publicradio.org.

Goethe, J. W. 1909. *Faust*. Trans. John Anster. London, Cassell.

Salick, E. C., and C. F. Auerbach. 2006. "From Devastation to Integration: Adjusting to and Growing from Medical Trauma." *Qualitative Health Research* 16(8): 1021–37.

Turner, D., and H. Cox. 2004. "Facilitating Posttraumatic Growth." *Health and Quality of Life Outcomes* 2(34).

Chapter 13

Bell, R. 2007. *Rethinking Justice: Restoring Our Humanity*. Lanham, MD: Lexington Books.

Berlinger, N. 2007. *After Harm: Medical Error and the Ethics of Forgiveness*. Baltimore, MD: Johns Hopkins University Press.

Bosk, C. 1979. *Forgive and Remember: Managing Medical Failure*. Chicago: University of Chicago Press.

Nouwen, H. 2007. *Beloved: Henri Nouwen in Conversation*. Cambridge: Wm. B. Eerdmans Publishing.

Pargament, K., K. Desai, and K. McConnel. 2006. "Spirituality: A Pathway to Posttraumatic Growth or Decline?" In *Handbook of Posttraumatic Growth: Research and Practice,* ed. L. Calhoun and R. Tedeschi, 121–37. New York: Lawrence Erlbaum Associates.

Chapter 14

Nouwen, H. 2007. *Beloved: Henri Nouwen in Conversation*. Cambridge: Wm. B. Eerdmans Publishing.

Sternberg, R. 2008. "Assessing Students for Medical School Admissions: Is It Time for a New Approach?" *Academic Medicine* 83(10): S105–S110.

Index